Never
Too
Late

# Never Too Late

## Your Guide to Safer Sex after 60

Shannon Dowler, MD

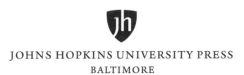

JOHNS HOPKINS UNIVERSITY PRESS

BALTIMORE

*Note to the Reader:* This book is not meant to substitute for medical care, and treatment should not be based solely on its contents. Instead, treatment must be developed in a dialogue between the individual and their physician. The book has been written to help with that dialogue.

*Drug dosage:* The author and publisher have made reasonable efforts to determine that the selection of drugs discussed in this text conforms to the practices of the general medical community. The medications described do not necessarily have specific approval by the US Food and Drug Administration for use in the diseases for which they are recommended. In view of ongoing research, changes in governmental regulation, and the constant flow of information relating to drug therapy and drug reactions, the reader is urged to check the package insert of each drug for any change in indications and dosage and for warnings and precautions. This is particularly important when the recommended agent is a new and/or infrequently used drug.

Johns Hopkins University Press
2715 North Charles Street
Baltimore, Maryland 21218
www.press.jhu.edu

Cataloging-in-Publication Data is available from the Library of Congress.

A catalog record for this book is available from the British Library.
ISBN: 978-1-4214-4633-2 (hardcover)
ISBN: 978-1-4214-4634-9 (paperback)
ISBN: 978-1-4214-4635-6 (ebook)

*Special discounts are available for bulk purchases of this book.*
*For more information, please contact Special Sales at specialsales@jh.edu.*

# Contents

# Never
# Too
# Late

———————

# You May Be Wondering Why I Have Called You Here Today

MARY WAS WIDOWED at a relatively young age—in her early 60s—following a decade of her husband's chronic illness. Her sex life had long since ceased and, after his death, she assumed she was done with love and intimacy. She felt blessed for what she had experienced in her marriage and certainly did not expect another chapter like the first. After a period of grieving, Mary settled into a solitary life, being a support to her adult children and grandchildren, gardening, and volunteering, until her world was turned topsy-turvy. She had not imagined dating again after losing her lifelong love. Then, in her mid-70s, she was asked out on a date. She could not imagine being romantic with another man. Not at her age. She had not had a date in decades. How did dating even work anymore?

Horrified, she vehemently rejected her pursuer for almost a month. He was persistent. She was intrigued. And thus unfolded a tale of two septuagenarians, both widowed, both discovering an unexpected world of dating and intimacy well into their Golden Years.

Mary's story is the new norm. Widowers, lifelong bachelors, and divorcées are finding more and more love, intimacy, and romance later and later in life. So much so that even the popular television show *The Bachelor* is launching a version for seniors looking for love. And there has never been a more opportune time to be in an intimate relationship or have sex. This applies to all consenting adults, but it is especially and uniquely true for the aging population. Who's in that lucky club, you might be wondering?

Let's be honest; if we're lucky, we will be part of the aging population because, as my dad used to say, "aging beats the alternative." (Granted, the darned pandemic threw cold water on some of the fun, but all hope is not lost—stick around for a deep dive on the impact of the pandemic in chapter 9.) For the purposes of our time together, I am talking about the 60-plus crowd, and here's the best news yet—you don't "age out" of sex. Older adults across the country and around the world are experiencing a sexual awakening that all the younger people who might be reading this book can only hope to one day enjoy. So, what makes today different from 1980 or even 2000?

Prior barriers to late-life sexuality have been lifted on many fronts over the past two decades. Hormonal regulation is achieved by clever, noninvasive methods of hormone replacement therapy and other technological advances. Sexual function is prolonged thanks to a class of highly effective pharmaceuticals as generics replace the historically cost-prohibitive brand names. More aging adults are living in closer proximity to each other in senior communities than at any other time in US history, and many are retiring at a younger age due to advances in financial planning, governmental incentives to save for retirement, as well as a generational shift in philosophy on work–life balance. Social media and smartphone applications can help you find a partner almost instantly, from the comfort of home. Whether you're seeking a casual connection on a weekend getaway or a brief work trip, or a longer-term partner, a companion is only a click away. It is a great time to be a 60-plus adult looking for love!

What could possibly go wrong?

Spoiler alert: So much can go wrong—but it doesn't have to.

Settle down in a comfy chair with your beverage of choice, and let's talk. You have opened the cover and turned the first page—now on to a no-holds-barred grown-up sex ed class. This is not a "how to" guide—I am not a sex therapist. This is not a rule book or morality primer. I am not here to serve up judgment.

Here's what I am here to do:

- Inform you about sexually transmitted diseases and infections (STDs), signs and symptoms to look out for, treatment options, and possible complications that can arise, and offer you ways to avoid contracting them.
- Share stories from my life and the experiences of other physicians, friends, and patients to show you real-life examples of what STDs are really like.
- Educate you about brand-new, hot-off-the-press risks to sexual intimacy that have arisen in recent years.
- Re-teach you things you once knew but forgot.
- Help you feel more comfortable talking about sex with your health care providers and sexual partners.
- Share facts, stats, and information that will make you the intimacy expert in the room.
- Raise awareness about the increasingly high rate of STDs plaguing the older demographic.
- Arm you with what you need to know to go forward in a safe and healthy sexual relationship.

In fact, I'm willing to bet that, by the end of this book, I will leave you far more "in the know" than your sophomoric grandkid who thinks they know it all. This book is not just for you sex revolution flower children from the 1960s who are leaping into the retired life. It's for all of you: swingers, doubters, abstainers, monogamists, adult children of aging parents, administrators of nursing homes and community living environments, preachers, teachers, and yes, even health care providers. If you are over 60, or know someone who is, I wager you are going to learn something in these pages that just may lead you to more intimacy and enjoyment in your later years than you'd thought possible.

If you are doubting the need for this book, let me take a minute to reassure you that the STD crisis in the United States is real. We are seeing year-over-year increases with no signs of relenting. If you look at the prevalence table (fig. I.1) from the US Centers for Disease Control and Prevention (CDC) and do not think you can wax poetic about who gets STDs and why we care, then keep reading. I can promise you, by the end of the book, you will be a lay expert and healthier for it.

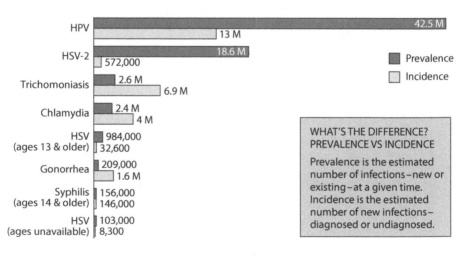

FIGURE I.1.
Prevalence and incidence of sexually transmitted infections in the United States, 2018. *Source:* cdc.gov

From a cost perspective alone, as a country we spend billions of dollars every year on treatment for sexually transmitted diseases, and the cost is continually growing. That is billions with a capital *B* followed by so many zeros! The graphic in figure I.2, also from the CDC, shows that the direct costs are $16 billion every year. Even more concerning, this estimate counts only direct costs. Imagine all the costs we do not even measure downstream and the impact on people's mental and physical health.

"Big deal," you may be saying as you pull out your golf clubs and head to the links. "Look at the statistics. That only happens to younger people. Older adults don't get STDs. Why do I need to know all this stuff?"

Trust me that you don't know what you don't know, and STDs are actually rising at a rapid rate in older adults. The national data are largely collected and focused on teens and young adults, which can make it more difficult to see the impact on older adults, but it is there and it is growing. Let's take a specific example. Chlamydia infection is

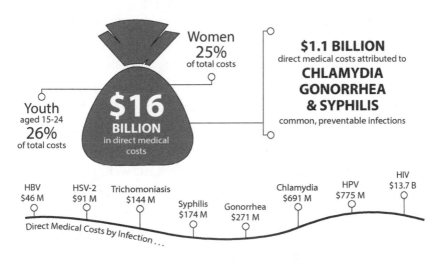

FIGURE I.2.
Direct costs of sexually transmitted infections in the
United States, 2018. *Source:* cdc.gov

from a bacterium you will learn a lot more about in chapter 4. Over the past two decades, chlamydia rates have gone from being essentially nonexistent for seniors to having rates double several times over.

Understanding the lay of the land never hurts, and this book will get you up to speed with an adults-only look at sex education. Here's the best news yet: this turn at sex ed is different than any you have had before. You are not in gym class with a bunch of awkward teenagers adorned with pimples and body odor or a well-meaning coach who is barely in control of the basics. It's just you and me—a physician who has treated STDs for over 20 years—and we are going to have a great time.

Who are the right students for this Best Ever Sex Ed Class? Anyone who is currently in a sexual relationship or seeking one in the near future should read this and, truthfully, it is good information for all ages. If you have friends exploring new relationships, this knowledge might help you help them navigate the potentially germ-laden waters they are swimming in. Perhaps you have a parent whom you'd like to better understand the sexual risks of later-in-life dating and you want to be able to provide answers if they have questions. Maybe you just need an excuse to buy this book to "help out a friend," but *you* are just really darned interested in getting up to speed on sex and STDs.

"Now wait just one second," those of you savvy with the vernacular of the current day might be yelling into the pages, "I thought we were supposed to call them STIs now, not STDs!" I will confess to being a little "old school." STD is the acronym of my youth. It is true that the controversy over the acronym is alive and well, and there will be a longer discussion of why in the next chapter. But to keep things simple, let's just stick with sexually transmitted diseases, or STDs, unless a particular study under discussion uses the alternate term.

This "Sex Ed on Steroids" class is for anyone interested in learning more about how to protect their bodies or how to understand what might be happening in the bodies all around you. It is okay if you are not now (and may never be) planning on jumping into the dating fray. Knowledge is power, and I am going to give you more than enough to feel comfortable in any conversation. Now, like any good teacher, I want to tell you a little bit about myself and explain why I am the best teacher for this particular class.

## My Story

First, let's talk about the elephant in the room. Why am I writing a book about people having sex in their 60s and beyond? Why am I writing a book about sex at all? (That's what my horrified teenagers are asking right now!) Let me tell you my story, and you will see how I came to be interested in and an expert on this topic, all the while balancing a full career as a health care leader and executive. Truthfully, STDs and sexual health have always been my "side gig," an extra-credit assignment, if you will, in an incredibly full and rewarding career. I am more than STDs, but when the cards are dealt, they are my favorite thing to study, treat, and talk about.

Since I am in full-on confession mode, I will tell you that I was not always very sex savvy. My journey to medicine and this health care niche was a path forged from broad experiences and exposures.

Much of what I learned about sex came from my Girl Scout troop, and often their knowledge was not exactly scientific. I remember being on a Girl Scout "lock-in" at Starmount Presbyterian Church. It was probably about three in the morning (one did not sleep at Girl Scout lock-ins unless you wanted to wake up with your face drawn on with markers or your hand submerged in warm water in the hopes that it would make you pee in the sleeping bag). I remember a group of us sitting in the choir room talking about boys. There was a giant chalkboard and when the topic came up about penises, foreskin, and circumcision, I had no idea what they were talking about. I could not wrap my brain around their descriptions. Luckily, one of my friends wasn't afraid to speak up and ask the question I had also been thinking:

"What the heck is a foreskin?" Another friend who had a brother and had seen a real-life penis (so was obviously the expert) tried to illustrate. What followed was a bizarre series of illustrations on the chalkboard as we all tried to understand what in the world this foreskin thing was about; I have since often wondered if we erased that chalkboard before the next choir rehearsal commenced.

Even though I wasn't the most educated on the topic, I was fascinated with sexual health and found myself increasingly interested as I became a teenager. (What teenager isn't interested in sex, you might be wondering?) As my Gold Award project for Girl Scouts my junior year of high school, I organized a day-long retreat for eighth-grade girls to teach them about dating safety, safe sex, and peer pressure. Even as an eleventh grader, I had witnessed and experienced some really tough things within my peer group: sexual harassment, sexual assault, unplanned pregnancy, and bullying, to name a few.

One night when I was in ninth grade, after I had gotten out of work at my part-time job at a local pizza place, I was taken to a remote road far out in the county with the promise of being "taught to drive a stick shift" by one of my coworkers whom I had a deep crush on. Once we got far away from any neighborhood, he demanded I perform oral sex or he would leave me on the side of that isolated country road in the dark, by myself. I remember shivering in the cold car and trying to decide if I was going to do what he asked or if worse things would happen if I stepped out of that car.

This was the 1980s and cell phones did not exist. I remember turning away, brokenhearted and terrified, and grabbing the door handle and yanking it open. I can still remember the stark fear I felt walking down that dirt road as the tires screeched away in the night. It was a while before his conscience forced him to return for me. He furiously drove me back to town and never spoke to me again.

My experiences were not unique. Most teenagers make errors in judgment, especially when it comes to love and dating, and many more suffer consequences from their actions. One friend scheduled an abortion when she discovered she was pregnant a month after her true love broke her heart and moved on. He had refused to use condoms, and she loved him, so she took the risk. She had no way to pay for it and came to me for help because I had a job. At the time, it was an impossible amount of money. I remember sitting down in the office with my boss, a wiry, hard-worn woman who chain smoked, filling the room with noxious vapor. I asked her for an advance on a paycheck. She was compassionate, but she declined. My friend ultimately gathered the money, but it resulted in a later termination of the pregnancy, and it was complicated by infection. She never told an adult or asked an adult for help.

Yet another friend spent an evening being rotated among the boys at a party where alcohol had flowed so freely that the ability to say "yes" or "no" was not possible. This was before "consent" meant actually saying "yes." In those days, consent often meant not saying "no," regardless of the lucidity of the person. There are not many women from my generation that can't put a #MeToo after their names. (For those of you not up on pop culture, there was a big social movement in the past decade where people acknowledged their previously suppressed history of sexual assault as a means to opening this topic for dialogue and understanding.)

So as a junior in high school, these topics of peer pressure, safe sex, and dating violence already resonated with me, and I wanted to make sure younger girls were equipped to navigate the difficult adolescent years with as much armor as possible. Having helped dear friends navigate dark days—making grown-up decisions with undeveloped frontal lobes—I believed that if I could shed some light for my younger sisters, then it was my job to do so.

It was a spring Saturday and the eighth-grade girls from troops around the city slowly arrived at the event and gathered in awkward groups. A few adult leaders stood together, laughing and talking. The day had been developed to offer a variety of topics, from peer pressure to pregnancy prevention (which was edgy content in the '80s). There were speakers from Planned Parenthood who helped us learn to put condoms on bananas and how to Say No. The peer pressure session included role-playing all the ways we could say "no" and still be "cool." To this day, the mantras we practiced in fits of giggles still come to mind when I'm forced to do things I don't want to do (namely chores). "Just because everyone else is doing it doesn't mean I have to" was a favorite.

Perhaps it was this day that became the spark of what would be a long career in education around sexual health, but at the time it just trying to help girls a little younger than me make it through adolescence happy and healthy.

I had flirted with the idea of being a veterinarian when I was a pre-teen. The books of James Herriot were on my bedside table at a young age, and his stories whispered to me. My first job, when I was 13, was at the vet hospital a mile from the house. I would ride my bike there on weekends and clean the cages and dog runs and feed the animals. I loved getting to assist the vet or go into surgery if my work was done early. I remember one dog with a growth on its side. The tech was busy tending to another animal, so the vet asked me to hold the dog while she incised his hairy side. Bursting from the incision was a thick, black, slug-like creature, wriggling at the end of the forceps. It was amazing! People with a weaker stomach may have been disgusted, but I was fascinated.

I always had two or three jobs in high school, and I became a receptionist at another vet hospital, which helped pay my bills. In college, I began thinking about life and the world and started questioning what I was supposed to be on earth to do. Where was I meant to go? What was I meant to do? Was being a vet my destiny? I knew that I had a love of medicine and helping the injured (whether human or canine), but I needed to make a definitive decision on which direction I wanted my career to go.

To help myself understand human medicine, I engrossed myself in it. I sought a college internship at Watauga Hospital and shadowed a gruff emergency room doctor, did a research project in the microbiology lab, and shadowed a kind pediatrician in his office. These experiences solidified the notion that taking care of people was my calling. In the emergency room, I saw so many patients who could not afford to treat their conditions. It was eye-opening and horrifying at the same time. There were countless people who could benefit from my medical education and eagerness to help people who had experienced less fortune than I had. So, I decided that summer I was going to take the path of human medicine to take care of those without wealth or access to health care. I would make a difference by taking care of the underserved.

Ready to graduate from Appalachian summa cum laude, I thought I was a hot commodity. I had received the top science award as a senior, I was president of the academic honor society Gamma Beta Phi, and I had received the Glaxo Women in Science Award. With confidence oozing from every pore, it is possible I was a little too full of myself. In my essay for my application to medical school, I quoted Stuart Smalley from *Saturday Night Live* and said the reason they should accept me to their medical school is because, "I'm good enough. I'm smart enough. And doggone it, people like me."

I was wait-listed.

The next year my application was far humbler, and I received early acceptance to East Carolina (now Brody) Medical School. Medical school was as difficult as you might imagine it would be, but once I got to the clinical years, my world expanded and my interest in sexual health was rejuvenated.

The country was still in the midst of the AIDS epidemic, and the crack cocaine phenomenon forced people off of the I-95 "drug belt" when they got too sick to continue on their journey. Many people infected with AIDS landed down east in North Carolina when I was a medical student. We provided them an option for medical treatment and cared for many of the men who were so young, beautiful, and dying.

The first case of syphilis I ever saw was on my pediatric rotation in my third year of medical school. A 12-year-old girl came in with a rash. The resident I was assigned to that day handed me a chart and said, "Here's a rash. Why don't you go in and take the history and then present her to me?"

The shy African American girl had not yet traversed puberty and sat in the corner of the room with her eyes downcast. I ran through the list of questions we had learned when faced with a rash. Any changes in soaps or detergents? Anyone else at home with the same thing? Any bites or new environmental exposures? What did the rash feel like? No itching. No pain. No changes in detergent. No medicines. No bug bites. No illness. I knew I was going to have to dig deeper if I was going to get to the diagnosis.

When I asked to see the rash, she turned up the palms of her hands. I saw dime-sized dark flat areas on her lighter-skinned palms.

"Hmmm," I said thoughtfully and unintelligently. "I will be right back with my attending," I announced, trying to sound perky. I did not want to scare the girl or unveil my ignorance. Completely unsure what it was, I presented the case to the resident and attending doctor. As I described the rash, their expressions immediately turned serious. The gravity was palpable. They taught me that there are few rashes that will occur on the palm and soles, and syphilis was the most likely contender in the absence of other signs of infection.

She was only 12, below the age of consent, so syphilis meant sexual abuse. The afternoon turned into a series of tests, calls to social services to report the case to Child Protective Services, tearful confessions, a painful shot of penicillin, and a case I would never forget. After myriad questions and much history taking, we ultimately learned her mother traded her daughter's body in exchange for drugs to feed her unrelenting crack cocaine addiction. My naïve heart wizened that day. While my father spent his career in Child Protective Services as a social worker, he had spared me the dark stories like these, and seeing this truth in the form of a sweet, young girl, wise beyond her years, imprinted in me a desire to protect those like her. I have often wondered what ultimately happened to that sweet girl with the upturned palms. Her quiet suffering, along with her abject poverty, spoke to me.

There were several areas of medicine that enticed me. Perhaps the most taunting muse was surgery. The crisp cleanliness of the OR and the opening of a human to reveal pink, pulsating tissue that could be excised to cure or alleviate illness and pain was like magic. Unfortunately, at that time, very few women were surgeons, and every surgery resident I worked with was already, or in the process of, a divorce. As I was a newlywed, this was frightening.

There were few women role models in surgery at that time. The one female surgery resident at my university was pregnant and was derided behind her back for not "holding her weight" with every other night call.

"You know the problem with taking call every other night?" the surgery residents would taunt medical students on rounds. "You miss half the cases!"

My decision to pursue family medicine after medical school was based on my desire to have the foundation to treat everyone, young and old, male and female, rich and poor. If I was totally honest, everything interested me. I could not just pick one. I loved something about all ages, but the children stole my heart. My first patient on a hospital ward was a young boy with prune belly syndrome, a rare condition where a person is born without any abdominal muscles, creating a compilation of other problems requiring many surgeries. This kid essentially grew up on the pediatric floor. His parents lived two hours away on a military base, and he spent days and weeks all alone in his hospital room. I would come in on weekends and stop by after long clinic days to play video games with him. When he was finally discharged home, I continued to wonder, worry, and think about him. I would often check to see if he had been readmitted. My desire to create a bond with him and support him was fueled by my anger at his parents for abandoning him there. After accessing all angles and contemplating which direction to go, I ultimately decided that family medicine provided the best opportunity to take care of all patients, work in a remote place, and still be able to have a comfortable work–life balance.

After "doing time" for four very hot years in the flatlands of Eastern North Carolina in medical school, we eagerly rushed up the mountain to a residency program awaiting us in Asheville, North Carolina. My family hails from rural Madison County (think *Cold Mountain*), so it's in my blood. My high school sweetheart and husband, Jared, was born and raised in the mountains of West Virginia. He felt a familiar comfort in the Appalachian Mountains that we have called home for over 20 years now.

During those years of residency, I worked grueling hours. On my ob-gyn rotation, 100- to 120-hour weeks were not uncommon. (This was before the work-hour restrictions were mandated to protect residents in training.) One day, after 13 straight days in the hospital, Jared picked me up after a 36-hour stretch without sleep so we could have a date and tour the Biltmore Estate, a grand historical home in the heart of Asheville. This was big money for us in those days, but it was a sunny day and we had hardly spent any time together. The last thing I remember was driving away from the hospital in wrinkled, tired scrubs before waking up hours later, pulling into our driveway in Black Mountain, a 20-minute drive. I rubbed my eyes in confusion.

"Sorry, I dozed off. Aren't we going to the Biltmore House?" I asked him.

Jared smiled and laughed.

"Dozed off? You've been asleep for hours. I didn't want to wake you," he explained.

"Honey, it's okay. Let's go!" I said, meaning it because that catnap restored me.

"Shannon, you slept all day. I toured the entire house, the grounds, and completed a wine tasting while you slept. I'm just glad no one saw you and called an ambulance. You were dead to the world!"

I had slept the deep slumber of the sleep-deprived in our compact car tucked in the shade of the parking lot. The significant others and spouses of medical students and residents have to learn to live incredibly independently, and Jared was no exception.

During my residency, opportunities to train in and learn sexual health continued to present themselves. One very busy night while I was on my ob-gyn rotation covering labor and delivery on the obstetrics service, we were forced to call security, and ultimately the police. A psychotic young man would not allow anyone to do a pelvic exam on his 12-year-old half-sister, who was 9 months pregnant and in labor with his baby. She was in early labor, but any labor for a girl this young is traumatic and overwhelming. She had not had any prenatal care, and certainly no childbirth classes, and she did not understand what was happening to her body. Wielding a knife and physically blocking us from her, he was convinced we were going to sexually assault her.

We were in the section of labor and delivery that was separated from the main delivery floor where women went before they were admitted to a bed. It was a small area just across the hallway from labor and delivery. As we waited for security to arrive, she was doubled over behind him, crying while he was ranting incoherently and waving a long, dirty hunting knife.

We took turns trying to gently approach.

"How about I just get your sister into the bed?" one nurse asked, with her hands held out calmly. "I won't touch her; I'll just help her get comfortable."

When security arrived, it was clear he was no stranger to law enforcement. Thankfully, he recognized defeat and just the sight of the police somehow pulled him out of his rage. His head drooped and he handed over his weapon. They bustled him away in handcuffs, and we descended on his terrified sister. Eventually, she went on to deliver a small, thankfully healthy baby.

Embedded forever in my memory is the vivid face of mental illness mixed with the stark reality of incest and sexual assault. She was below the age of consent and her baby would be given to foster care unless a family member could demonstrate the ability to care for the infant. The despair I felt that night knowing that this tiny new life might very well follow a similar path as generations of backwoods culture isolated in the many pockets of Appalachia changed me. Eye-opening experiences like this as a young doctor further influenced my desire to protect the vulnerable.

Sexual abuse in children is an all-too-common and grossly under-reported phenomenon in this country. In the late 1990s, it was estimated that 10% to 15% of children experienced sexual abuse by a family member, with 2% experiencing intercourse. Sexual abuse as a child correlates to ongoing challenges for many men and women. An article from 2013 in *The Atlantic* explains it well:

> Ninety-five percent of teen prostitutes and at least one-third of female prisoners were abused as kids. Sexually abused youth are *twice as likely* to be arrested for a violent offense as adults, are at twice the risk for lifelong mental health issues and are twice as likely to attempt or die from teen suicide. The list goes on. Incest is the single biggest commonality between drug and alcohol addiction, mental illness, teenage and adult prostitution, criminal activity, and eating disorders. Abused youths don't go quietly into the night. (emphasis added)

The experiences from my adolescence, college internships, medical school, and residency pointed me to a career in public health. I chose extra rotations during residency in the health department STD clinic and got a paid job moonlighting there during my fellowship year. A week after completing my fellowship, I accepted my first "real doctor" job and joined the health department as a full-time family doctor, caring for pregnant women, children, and adults, with one half-day a week—Wednesday morning—specially carved out to staff the STD clinic, where I continue to work today. Many of the stories I will share in this book are from my experiences in this active clinic.

I like to tell newcomers to the Asheville area, "We have it all." Beautiful views, whitewater, amazing food, and rich culture are just a few of its features. As a tourist destination, we attract visitors from all over the country; as such, our STD rates have been more like that of a big urban city than a sleepy mountain community. As travelers come and go, they often leave behind sightless, soundless infections that work their way through the community. It is a wondrous place to live and love, but you might just bring home more than you bargained for!

I started my career as a family doctor with time in the STD clinic, and while my 20-year career as a physician has taken increasingly larger roles into state and national leadership, I continue to dedicate time at the STD clinic, where I am professionally my happiest. But, enough about me. It's time to talk about you!

## CHAPTER 1

# Sex
# in the
# Twenty-First Century

Gotta be safe, cause sex has gotten risky,
No shame being a freak and getting a little frisky!

## Are Sexually Transmitted Diseases
## and Infections Really That Big a Deal?

THE SEXUAL REVOLUTION that began in the 1960s challenged social norms and traditional concepts, promoted acceptance, and liberated individuals from sexual repression. It effectively transformed society and how we, in the United States, thought about sex. Today, those same people are helping us see that sexual exploration in the Golden Years remains as vigorous as it was in the 1960s. Unfortunately, along with increased sexual activity comes the risk of sexually transmitted diseases.

It's a common misconception that the younger generation is the *only* group susceptible to infection. Adolescents and young adults make up only 25% of the sexually active population, but they are diagnosed with over 50% of the sexually transmitted infections, so they are definitely top contenders. Surprisingly though, seniors over the

A few lines of lyrics from my YouTube educational rap video "STDs Never Get Old," written by me, appear at the beginning of each chapter. See the appendix for the full lyrics.

age of 55—baby boomers—are actually one of the fastest-growing demographics contracting STDs. The children who explored free love at Woodstock and sexual promiscuity at Studio 54 are now thriving in retirement communities, with Viagra and Cialis in their pockets and nothing but time on their hands. Without the threat of pregnancy looming overhead, seniors are engaging in unprotected sex at an alarming rate. According to a study published by Athena Health, seniors have the lowest condom use of any population. This makes sense if the only reason you use a condom is to prevent pregnancy, but barrier methods (forms of contraception that create a physical barrier between the male's sperm and the female's egg) are also critical to preventing unwanted infections by blocking the exchange of body fluids, and all signs point to the reality that seniors aren't using them.

Sexually transmitted diseases and infections are at an all-time high in the United States, with increases year after year for the past decade and no sign of relenting. According to the World Health Organization, more than 1 million sexually transmitted infections (STIs) are acquired *every day* worldwide. Each year, in the United States, there are an estimated 376 million new infections with one of four STDs: chlamydia, gonorrhea, syphilis, or trichomoniasis. (This is a great time to consider your need for sex ed: how familiar are you with all of these incredibly common infections?) More than 500 million people are estimated to have genital infection with herpes simplex virus. More than 290 million women have a human papillomavirus (HPV) infection. The Centers for Disease Control and Prevention (CDC) says that the rapid increase in people contracting STDs must be confronted. And I agree.

Jonathan Mermin, MD, director of the CDC National Center for HIV/AIDS, viral hepatitis, STD, and TB prevention, stated, "STDs are a persistent enemy, growing in number, and outpacing our ability to respond." The CDC reported that in 2017 nearly 2.3 million cases of chlamydia, gonorrhea, and syphilis were reported in the

United States. That is the highest number ever recorded for these diseases. Since 2015, STD rates have gone up considerably and consistently: gonorrhea is up 56%, primary and secondary syphilis up 74%, chlamydia 19%, and congenital syphilis 279%—yes, 279%!

There have been many advances, including rapid lab testing and our ability to more quickly make an accurate diagnosis, improved treatments and tolerable treatment regimens, preventive breakthroughs like vaccinations, and overall increased access to health care across the country, in all age groups. Despite these changes, we are consistently watching rates increase across a variety of STDs and age groups, not just in the United States but around the world. A snapshot of STD rates in 2018 from the CDC website is given in figure 1.1.

Infection rates for sexually transmitted diseases keep climbing among Americans 55 and older. The *Daily Mail* in the United Kingdom reported that the number of STDs among the 50 to 70 age group soared by 38% between 2013 and 2016. The CDC published its *Morbidity and Mortality Weekly Report* stating, "More than 2 million U.S.

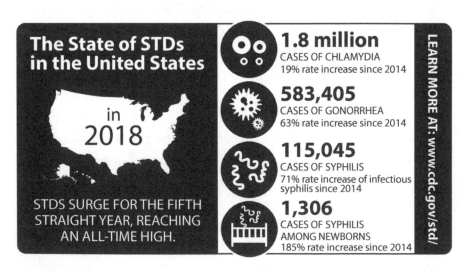

FIGURE 1.1.
The state of sexually transmitted diseases in the United States, 2018.
*Source:* cdc.gov

baby boomers are infected with hepatitis C—accounting for more than 75% of all American adults living with the virus." But hepatitis is only one of the many diseases threatening the older community.

Athena Health's website states, "Between 2014 and 2017, diagnosis rates for herpes simplex, gonorrhea, syphilis, chlamydia, hepatitis B, and trichomoniasis rose 23% in patients over the age of sixty." Some STDs can be fatal. Human papillomavirus (HPV) can lead to cervical, anal, penile, and head and neck cancers, and we all know the threat that HIV poses.

It may be troubling to think that Grandma and Grandpa are at serious risk for HIV and AIDS, but it is the reality we live in. The CDC reported that in 2016, nearly half of people in the United States living with HIV were aged 50 and older. In 2017, one in six new HIV diagnoses were people over the age of 55. Older patients represent the largest increase in treatments of STDs seen by health care providers' offices (fig. 1.2).

At the end of 2016, only 60% of people over 50 with HIV were virally suppressed (that means they are not as infectious and are less likely to spread the disease), and the CDC estimates that 1 in 10 people over 50 infected with HIV do not know they have the infection. So, the 40%

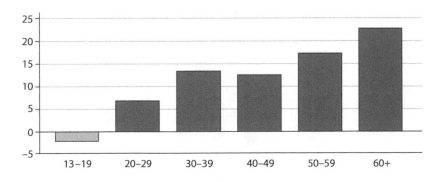

FIGURE 1.2.
Between 2014 and 2017, more older people sought in-office treatment of sexually transmitted diseases than any other age group.
*Source:* Data from athenahealth.com

who are not virally suppressed and the 10% who don't know they are infected are actively spreading the infection—whether they know it or not—if they are not using condoms 100% of the time (fig. 1.3). And, let's face it, very few people are able to use condoms 100% of the time.

I can tell you that in North Carolina, a state with a relatively large number of older adults, we have seen five consecutive years of end-over-end increases in both the 50–64 and the 65+ age categories in chlamydia, gonorrhea, *and* syphilis. If you look at the national data available on the CDC website, you will see the same trends. In the chlamydia graphic in figure 1.4, you see the rates increased year-over-year since 2015, with a 100% increase in men 55–64 and a 75% increase in men over 65. While women showed slightly slower rate increases, women often have silent and asymptomatic infections and are more likely to go undiagnosed. For gonorrhea, on the other hand, you see the rates increase on the magnitude of 100% to 160% for the same time frame for both age groups and in both men and women (fig. 1.5).

The graph in figure 1.6 shows the rate of syphilis growth in older adults. You can see the same pattern of increases from 100% to nearly 160% for both men and women in both age groups. The last graph, in figure 1.7, demonstrates the steady year-over-year rise of HIV

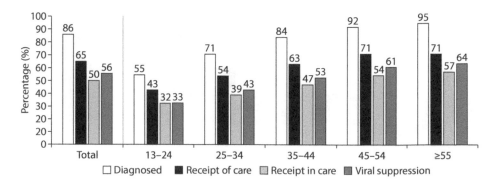

FIGURE 1.3.
Stages of HIV care by age, 2018. *Source:* Centers for Disease Control and Prevention. *HIV Surveillance Report 2016*; vol 28.

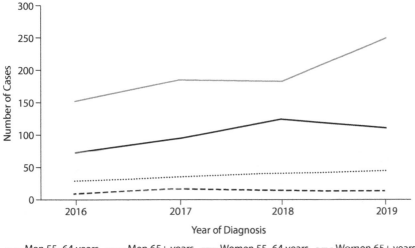

FIGURE 1.4.
Newly diagnosed chlamydia cases in North Carolina for men
and women ages 55–64 and 65+ between 2016 and 2019.
*Source:* North Carolina Electronic Disease Surveillance (data as of July 6, 2021)

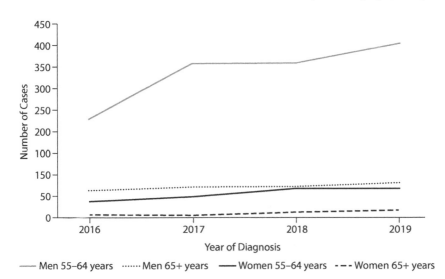

FIGURE 1.5.
Newly diagnosed gonorrhea cases in North Carolina for men
and women ages 55–64 and 65+ between 2016 and 2019.
*Source:* North Carolina Electronic Disease Surveillance (data as of July 6, 2021)

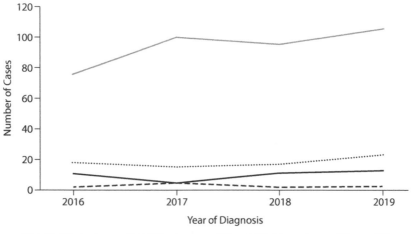

FIGURE 1.6.
Newly diagnosed early syphilis cases in North Carolina for men
and women ages 55–64 and 65+ between 2016 and 2019.
*Source:* North Carolina Electronic Disease Surveillance (data as of July 6, 2021)

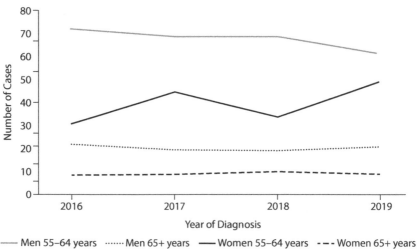

FIGURE 1.7.
Newly diagnosed HIV cases in North Carolina for men
and women ages 55–64 and 65+ between 2016 and 2019.
*Source:* North Carolina Electronic Disease Surveillance (data as of June 28, 2021)

infection in older adults. This is only categorized in the CDC data as 55+, but you see dramatic increases in people living with HIV from year to year since 2014, in both men and women. These annual increases follow relatively flat numbers for the entire decade before. Something changed after 2014 and has persisted. The data do not lie. The number of sexually transmitted infections in older adults is climbing across the board.

Are you wondering why I am not showing you the same graph with herpes?

Unfortunately, in the United States, not all STDs are reportable. Reportable infections must be shared from the health care provider's office to the local health department, which then shares it with state public health, which then shares the data with the CDC. The CDC makes this data publicly available, so anyone interested in these public health issues can go mine the data. In the United States, we focus on reporting on the infections that we can track and cure when they are treatable. We also track treatable but incurable diseases to diminish or prevent their spread. Unfortunately, we only have the ability to track the data across the country and see these trends for infections that are reportable. We do not measure or track herpes, HPV, trichomonas, or *Mycoplasma genitalium* (Mgen), among others. (If some of these are new names for you, we are only just beginning. Buckle up and keep on reading!) We are seeing across-the-board rates increasing for every age group and almost every sexually transmitted infection that we monitor.

Men and women who have not been "on the market" in 40 or more years are grossly unprepared to navigate this new sexual milieu. The last time they were finding new partners there were far fewer STDs present at much lower rates. Widows and widowers, surprised to fall in love again in their 70s and 80s, may have never even heard of trichomonas, human papillomavirus, or *Mycoplasma genitalium*. There is also a marked difference in the sexual education these baby boomers received—or didn't receive—growing up. Fifty years ago, schools were not educating students about sex and STDs the way they currently are. And the ones that did offer some sort of sexual health education contained what is now considered outdated information that has changed significantly over several decades. The senior community has limited education about STDs, the risks they command, the symptoms they present, preventive measures, or treatment responses because there simply wasn't a widespread public health emphasis on safe sex.

This phenomenon is global. In 2018, ABC News in Australia stated, "Straight male baby boomers are less likely than younger men to use condoms or know much about sexual health, leaving them vulnerable to infections." Family Planning New South Wales did a study and reported that "men aged 50 or older were less likely to use condoms and more likely than younger men to think that condoms reduced sexual interest." If you ask someone in their 70s or 80s if they used a condom when they were sexually active in their youth, chances are the answer will be "no." The need for condoms was not fully understood or appreciated in the mid-1900s. Though most baby boomers were sexually active in the 1950s, '60s, and '70s, they were not receiving the proper sexual education from their parents, who came of age in a sexually ignorant era. Sigmund Freud opposed condoms, stating that they cut down on sexual pleasure, many feminist groups opposed male-controlled methods of contraception, and the Roman Catholic Church affirmed its opposition to all contraceptives, including the condom.

Those who did use condoms in their earlier days were often doing so as a source of contraception, not to prevent sexually transmitted infections. It wasn't until the AIDS epidemic of the 1980s that condoms were looked at as a tool for safer sex. Many baby boomers were already married or settled down by the 1980s, so they didn't (and some still don't) comprehend the importance of condoms to prevent sexually transmitted diseases because it didn't apply to them. Now these same people are engaging in active sex lives in their later years when pregnancy is no longer a possibility due to menopause, but they are still harboring the same mindset toward condoms. A study by sex researchers at Indiana University found that in the United States, condom use was lowest among men 50 and older. The AARP website has numerous blogs about the importance of condom use in older adults and recognizes that there is a need to improve.

So baby boomers are more sexual than ever, STD rates are at their highest on record, and seniors over 55 are the fastest-growing demographic contracting STDs; yet many baby boomers don't fully understand the need for condoms (most of them are not even using protection), they are not being screened properly, and they have virtually no sexual education about the risks associated with the STDs that they are regularly exposing themselves to. What could possibly go wrong?

In addition to the known infections that are transmitted sexually, new players continue to arrive on the scene. While I will admit that I get really excited when I hear about a new STD (more things to rhyme about!), it is not a good sign for those of you out there having new partners. Have you heard of *Mycoplasma genitalium*? If not, read on. Did you know Ebola and the Zika virus are sexually transmitted? It is not every day a new sexually transmitted infection is identified. As a matter of fact, while this book was in the editing process, we have a burgeoning new infection we have learned can be transmitted sexually—monkeypox. Of course, some are as old as time. Here's a good dinner table fact for you. Herpes dates back 3 million years when it crossed species, according to a study in *Virus Evolution*. New technology has allowed us to identify species we did not know existed before and to understand more fully the many ways they can travel from one person or animal to the next.

Syphilis has been troubling genitals for hundreds of years and is still going strong. In the late 1400s, a wave of syphilis plagued Europe, effectively putting the disease on the map. Syphilis cases in the United States have been reported as early back as the sixteenth century and are theorized to have been brought to the US by European explorers (more on this in chapter 2). Other infections have likely been in existence longer than the doctors of their day knew. According to *Encyclopedia Britannica*, syphilis and gonorrhea were long thought to be one disease. Real progress in characterizing them did not occur until the early twentieth century, when their different causative microorganisms were identified and reliable diagnostic tests were developed.

To really pile on the problem and disrupt your sleep tonight, in addition to the myriad STDs we do not track and the new ones we keep discovering, well-known bacteria (like gonorrhea that causes "the clap") are developing resistance to antibiotics. The first fully drug-resistant case of gonorrhea hit the United Kingdom in 2019. That means we literally do not have an antibiotic tested and approved to treat the resistant strains of the infection. Our arrogance that we can effectively treat and cure infections is rapidly waning. COVID-19 has gone a long way to helping society see the menace that a rapidly evolving and changing organism can be in only a matter of months. It can take decades to discover, test, and approve a new drug, and many STDs are developing resistance faster than we can outsmart them.

Relatively speaking, the aging population barely hits the radar. Public health eyes are focused on younger adolescents and adults for prevention efforts. And that makes some sense. Baby boomers aren't going to get pregnant and transmit a devastating infection to a baby. They are less likely to be a sex worker, spreading infection widely from street corner to street corner. But our bodies are still our greatest gift and, frankly, our most vulnerable possession. Our bodies become more susceptible as we age. While the CDC is off stomping out the big fires, your health deserves the focus as well. You owe it to your body to be thoughtful if you are entering into a new relationship or continuing an open relationship. Even if today you are not planning to become intimate with someone new, who knows what tomorrow will hold? Better to get up to speed now. As they say, better to be safe than sorry! With rates increasing year-over-year in the aging demographic, there is no question that your risk (or your best friend's, brother's, or mom's risk) is increasing by the day.

### You Say Po-tay-toe, I Say Po-tah-toe: Which Acronym Is Right, STD or STI?

We talked about this in the introduction, and I promised to unpack the Great Acronym Debate. Which is it, you may be asking, sexually transmitted diseases (STDs) or sexually transmitted infections (STIs)? This is a point of great controversy and angst in the sexual health world, and it really comes down to three things: stigma, semantics, and money.

There are many who believe that the stigma attached to a "disease" is far worse for people. They might avoid diagnosis and treatment out of fear of having a disease, whereas "infection" is generally perceived as more transitory and time-limited and less severe—would you rather be "diseased" or "infected"?

There is also the semantics controversy. It is true that some sexually transmitted bacteria and viruses cause infections that do not proceed to disease. For instance, a brief bout with chlamydia urethritis (that's when a male has the infection in his urinary tract) is cured with one dose of antibiotics. Yet the very same sexually transmitted bacteria can proceed to pelvic inflammatory disease (a more serious and persistent infection in women), which you will learn about in chapter 4.

"Infection" suggests a time-limited, transitory state, whereas "disease" suggests a longer-term problem, right? Sort of (or "ish" as my teen niece, Ellie, says). Herpes infection, caused by a virus, is

lifelong for most people and causes recurrent bouts of painful ulcers on the mucosa (typically the mouth or genitals). Is that an infection or a disease? Or both? HIV can now be effectively suppressed
with a regimen of antiviral drugs, so a person has no detectable viral
load. Then are these infections or diseases? The truth is, there is a
continuum. "STI" advocates say "STD" comes with an unnecessary
stigma. I get that—who wants to have a disease? Most of us would
pick infection with the assumption it can be cured. Having said that,
culturally, I believe we are a long way from anything sex-related not
being stigmatized in this country regardless of what acronym you
use.

At the end of the day, it all comes down to money. Doesn't it always? "STD" advocates also say that to rebrand entire government
disease control and communicable disease branches would cost tax-
payers hundreds of millions—possibly even billions—of dollars, and
many of the infections do lead to diseases. Increasingly around the
world, the "STI" acronym is being used. This is true of the World
Health Organization, and our recently released National Strategic
Plan is dubbed the STI plan. In 2021, for the first time, the historical,
highly lauded (by some of us, anyway) "STD Guidelines," published
by the CDC STD Branch, were published as the "STI Guidelines."
Game. Set. Match.

I say, why can't we all just get along? Whether you say STI or STD
or cover all the bases and say STD/I, it really doesn't matter to me. The
bottom line is, we don't want you to get any of them!

## Why the Older Population? Why Now?

There are a handful of key contributors to how we got to this place of
rising rates of STDs in the older population: sociocultural changes,
the inevitability of biology fails with age, and, ironically, advances in
technology. Each one alone could certainly contribute to a blip in the
radar, but together they are the cause of this rather drastic spike

contributing to the evolving STD epidemic in older adults. We will delve deeply into these topics in the coming chapters.

A community that has been in the news for years for its staggering STD rates is The Villages, in Florida. According to the US Census Bureau, the Villages is home to almost 80,000 seniors; it spreads across 65 miles and contains more than 50 golf courses. The Villages is the fastest-growing US city for the second year in a row, and STD cases are climbing as well. AARP says, "In Central Florida, where The Villages and other retirement communities sprawl across several counties, reported cases of syphilis and chlamydia increased 71% among those fifty-five and older."

I know a great number of people who live and play in retirement communities and nursing homes, and they all have stories. If you go on the Internet and google "STDs in the elderly," you will find countless stories about retirement community sex scandals. There are urban legends galore, ranging from scrunchies on golf carts to indicate partner preference, to sex parties and free-love swingers' clubs. Did I just say scrunchies? The rumors suggest that displaying different colored hair ties (known to youngsters as scrunchies) or loofahs (a type of sponge for cleaning and exfoliating) can help denote if you are interested in sex with a man, woman, or both. True story: As my mom had more and more trouble finding her Subaru Outback in parking lots in the mountains of North Carolina, she took to putting loofahs on her roof rack to make her car stand out . . . that is, until I told her she was advertising her sexual preferences for everyone to see! There are plenty of articles that pop up on the subject when you do a Google search, which led me to believe that there is some truth in the stories, even if it's not as prevalent as the Internet would have us believe. Are the many-splendored tales of The Villages fact or fiction? Good or bad? Maybe it is a little of both. I decided to find out for myself. I connected with a delightful woman who lives in The Villages who was recently widowed. She offered some interested insights.

"When you go to the square, you can pick out the women and couples who are out for a good time."

I asked her to validate the rumor of "the golf cart scrunchy."

She laughed and said, "Yes, now that is true! Maybe that's why I stopped playing golf!"

Whether all the stories out there reflect real-world circumstances, I am in no position to verify; to be honest, I kind of hope they do. We should all age so enthusiastically! The cultural shift in our country toward communal retirement living creates abundant opportunities for the spread of infections. Dial back to your college days. Remember dorm life—people living in close proximity, pheromones oozing from the walls. Now imagine what college would have been like without the actual college part. Suddenly there are no classes to go to, no exams to cram for, no work responsibilities, and no risk of getting—or getting someone else—pregnant. Ch-ch-ch-ching! It is, literally, all the fun of college without any of the hassles!

Skilled nursing home facilities have long navigated the awkward phenomenon of sexual activity in elderly patients in long-term nursing care for a variety of reasons. For instance, men and women suffering from frontal lobe dementia are often disinhibited and have increased sexual desires without the social inhibition of the frontal lobe (simply put, if it itches, scratch it). The concerns of these administrators are largely over competency and consent and avoiding any possibility of abuse or neglect, which can be a difficult balance while respecting patient autonomy. What's wrong with consensual intimacy? Retirement communities differ from skilled nursing in that they bring together independent and highly functioning adults enjoying preserved good health who may be eager to engage in sexually gratifying encounters and rediscovered intimacy but who are ill prepared for the consequences of their newfound sexual reality. Intimacy creates a unique vulnerability.

An example would do.

I was working at the urgent care not that long ago when a well-dressed woman in her late 60s (let's call her "Zelda") came in with the complaint of vaginal discharge. She did not want to go to her primary care doctor because she was uncomfortable sharing her recent sexual encounter and preferred to keep the records separate. She had spent the weekend with a few very good friends at a cabin in the mountains where they had a lovely time soaking in a hot tub with wine, fellowship, and shared sex toys. They were also stewing in chlamydia, as it turned out.

"They all seemed clean," she remarked with a furrow in her brow. (Don't worry, if you have forgotten about chlamydia, you are going to get to know it well in chapter 4.)

Zelda is a perfect example of how looks can be deceiving, and you should never judge a book by its cover. You can be sure that people of all colors, races, ethnicities, sizes, shapes, and social classes can be harboring an STD and not know it (fig. 1.8).

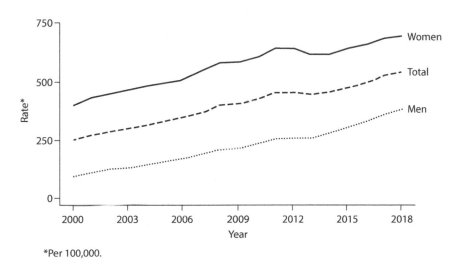

*Per 100,000.

FIGURE 1.8.
Rates of reported cases of chlamydia by sex in the United States
from 2000 through 2018. *Source:* cdc.gov

Zelda's story was actually the inspiration for one of my STD limericks:

> "Looks Aren't Everything"
> Dear Chlamydia, your timing's not great,
> But it sure was a fabulous date!
> The fella looked clean
> (if you know what I mean)
> Perhaps PID's just a matter of fate.

Zelda was treated at the clinic, and a disease control form was faxed over to the health department. Oh yes, this is a reportable disease, so it goes to a nurse at the health department whose job it is to make sure the patient is adequately treated and all potential partners are contacted. We work incredibly hard in public health to protect the privacy of the people we care for, but reportable diseases fall into a unique category. While people can always lie or share incomplete information, the hope is that people will share their infection information to protect the health of those around them. Unfortunately, there are not enough health care dollars to meaningfully track partners of people diagnosed with chlamydia and gonorrhea, but if you get hepatitis B or C, HIV/AIDS, or syphilis, you can count on a visit and all your partners getting contacted.

So, Zelda had to call all her friends stewing in the same hot tub (as well as any other recent sexual partners) and tell them they needed antibiotics. This can be really hard for people to do because of the stigma that is attached to sexually transmitted infections. If we could think of them like strep throat or influenza, you might feel bad for giving something to a friend, but you probably would not feel a deep sense of shame. To make the "partner contact" easier, I suggest that my patients who cannot imagine calling someone take a picture of the disease notification card, text it to people who were potentially exposed, and ask them to see a health care provider for treatment.

Zelda completed her contacts and was instructed on sex toy hygiene to prevent re-infection. It was kind of a bummer end to what she reported was a great weekend, and it would have been totally avoidable if they had all previously gotten appropriate STD screening tests and received treatment.

## Gender Identity and Sexual Orientation

Another phenomenon in American culture over the past decade is an increasing acceptance of gender fluidity and an openness to nonbinary gender identification. You may be asking, what does that even mean? Binary sexual identification is clearly defined as being one or the other: male or female. Nonbinary refers to the many people for whom it is not that simple. Nonbinary people often identify as both sexes. They are both masculine and feminine and don't want to be forced into choosing one or the other. They choose to use pronouns like "they" and "them."

In addition to nonbinary gender identity creating new patterns of sexual behavior, there is an increasing tolerance and acceptance for sexual identity variations beyond the typical "gay" or "straight" line. There is homo-, hetero-, pan-, a-, and bi-sexuality to consider. This changes our sexual habitat and, combined with gender fluidity, creates a very different worldview for many people who have lived relatively closeted lives. If you are like my mom, you might struggle with some of the new terms. Change isn't always easy.

I will be honest—sometimes I step in it myself when talking to my kids about a friend who I knew for a decade as a "she" who is now a "he" or a "they." It's worth trying to comprehend, so I'm including some common definitions to get you up to speed. Here are some very basic terms related to sexual orientation and gender identity:

*Asexual:* having no sexual attraction to others
*Bisexual:* sexually attracted to both male and female genders
*Cisgender:* birth gender and gender identity are the same

*Gender binary:* the belief that there are only two genders and everyone fits into one of the two

*Gender nonconforming:* nontraditional gender expression/identity

*Heterosexual:* sexually attracted to someone of a different gender

*Homosexual:* sexually attracted to someone of the same gender

*Nonbinary:* identifying as both a male and a female, masculine and feminine

*Pansexual:* sexually attracted to all genders

*Transgender:* someone has transitioned from one gender to another

If this is something you would like to understand more about, there are countless resources available for free on the Internet. For additional definitions, consider this resource: https://www.its pronouncedmetrosexual.com/2013/01/a-comprehensive-list-of -lgbtq-term-definitions/.

I like to think of myself as unusually enlightened, especially when it comes to matters of sexuality. After all, it is core to my career. I learned the hard way that we never stop learning. When I was in Denver, Colorado, at a national conference in 2015, I was having lunch with a colleague and good friend, Dr. Rhett Brown. We were discussing transgender health issues. He had been an early advocate and specialist for transgender health care. Patients travel hours to see him, across state lines, because physicians trained and knowledgeable in this field have been relatively limited until recently.

My good friend, who was also a church pastor, had a child who was born female and, at the age of 14, decided to transition to a male. She (now he) was undergoing heavy hormone therapy to stunt puberty and was considering "top" surgery (a bilateral mastectomy to remove both breasts). It's not that I disagreed with this type of surgery, or the benefits of helping someone transition into their "true" self, but I shared my concern with Rhett that I was really struggling, as a physician, with the idea of an adolescent going through a permanent gender-confirming process. I was worried that such a life-altering, irreversible decision at such a young age could be something they might mature to regret.

Rhett looked me in the eye and with his incredibly patient and kind voice said, "Shannon, when did you know you were a girl?"

I immediately saw his point. And, of course, he was right. Rhett is always right!

I knew from a very young age that I was a girl, not because someone told me, but because I just was. Sure, I was a touch of a "tomboy"; when the chores were distributed, my sister picked polishing silver and I eagerly donned work gloves and cleaned the gutters and mowed. But there was never any doubt I was a girl. This core understanding has helped me translate an important concept into practice as a physician. Key to all of us excelling in our professions is cycles of continuous learning and improvement and addressing and combating our implicit biases.

I share my own progression as a physician in understanding and accepting gender fluidity not so much as it relates to STDs but as it relates to what is very new thinking from a sociocultural standpoint. I could devote an entire chapter to the very real heath disparities that sexual minorities experience, but that is for another day.

### The Bottom Line

I am confident that by the end of this book, you will be the life of the bridge party, golf course, or book club, showering your friends with newfound wisdom and insights, and maybe even doling out relationship advice. Perhaps you will feel empowered to corner a friend you know has been making risky choices and make sure they have the information they need. Maybe you have a parent you are concerned about, and now you feel more comfortable broaching the topic. Or maybe, just maybe, you will feel secure in all that you have learned and decide you're ready to join the party!

## CHAPTER 2

# The Biology of Aging and Sexually Transmitted Diseases

Quick to the point, to the point I'm making,
Lubrication's key and you know I'm not faking.

GEORGE USED TO LOVE attending the downtown music festival every summer. It was the highlight of his year and something he looked forward to almost as much as Christmas. As an elderly man in his 80s, he lived in a senior subsidized housing high-rise in the heart of downtown, so the festival meant a weekend of free entertainment and joviality right in his "backyard." It was four days of bands, food trucks on every corner, and a street party that reminded him of his one Mardi Gras venture many years before.

George also loved the music festival for another very specific reason. Every year he would save up his money and "splurge" during the festival on a little gift for himself—and it was a gift that just kept giving. For the three years that I knew George, in the week following the festival he would shuffle down to the STD clinic, only a few blocks from his home, his eyes cast down with a subtle smile playing at the edges of his mouth and declare, with just a hint of pride, "Doc, I'm drippin'." For George, his retained vigor so late in life was an easy trade-off for the occasional dose of gonorrhea.

The biology of the human body is an ever-changing thing. As we grow and age, our bodies undergo both obvious and subtle changes. As I have traversed menopause and observed my children navigate adolescence, I am awed by the ways our internal workings affect our very form and function as humans. The media and younger generations like to poke fun at the idea of Senior Sex, complicated by wrinkles and arthritis, but the truth is that it is a celebration to be able to include intimacy in your aging life. At the same time, it is also important that we acknowledge some of the changes in the body with age that can impact sexual functioning and, ultimately, lead to acquisition of sexually transmitted infections. In this chapter we will review the aging body, understand the evolution of drug resistance, and take a quick look at STDs in history.

### "Haters"
The young, they may turn a cold shoulder.
Their censure gets louder and bolder.
We should all be so lucky
To be amorous and plucky
With intimacy as we get older!

### Erectile Dysfunction

The market is full of "fixes" for cosmetic things like wrinkles, joint pain, and erectile dysfunction. Many men, like George, navigate their senior years without the need of additional support for sexual function, but the incidence of all forms of sexual dysfunction increases with age. What was once a hopeless, and for many, shameful condition, now has an "easy button" for many men in the form of medications to increase the much-needed blood flow to create a functional erection. There are numerous reasons why a man may experience a decrease in sexual function with age and, interestingly, not all men do (as opposed to menopause, which leaves no woman behind!).

A combination of chronic illnesses and the medications used to treat these conditions contributes to many men losing full sexual functioning later in life. Treatments for prostate cancer and what is now being looked on as overly aggressive screening and procedural treatment have contributed to the number of men in the senior generation experiencing challenges with erectile function. Even for men who are not candidates for the medications, including such household names as Viagra and Cialis, there are an array of mechanical fixes at your friendly urologist's office, like pumps and penile implants. Indeed, hope is not lost.

The advent of medications like Viagra and Cialis revolutionized sexual function and performance. Early on, those medications were cost prohibitive for many patients as they would sell for $10 a pill, leaving many patients to hold on to them for special occasions but not consistently enjoy their sexuality. But generic producers have resulted in dramatically reduced costs, and many insurance plans now cover them. Insurance coverage of these medications was quite controversial in the years prior to the Affordable Care Act, as many insurance companies would cover the cost of erectile-enhancing drugs but not the cost of contraceptives. Even without a health care provider's prescription, in our modern era, enhanced access to these drugs occurs for many patients through international online access or simply traveling to countries that do not require a prescription. My parents very generously bought a "family cruise" for Christmas a few years ago and every port we stopped in had pharmacies with huge signs, scrawled in red, advertising their prices for erectile dysfunction medications without a prescription. Access to pharmaceuticals to treat erectile dysfunction is more widespread now than ever, but that means it's often without the counsel or input of a physician. "Male health clinics" often offer testosterone injections, and many online clinics offer treatments without following important markers for prostate cancer or performing important physical exam components.

These "easy buttons" may be great in the moment, but they are not ideal for a couple of key reasons that I hope you will consider if you or your friends are securing these medications through nontraditional channels. First, by eliminating the office visit, a patient is losing out on timely and important guidance, and opportunities for screening for infections related to a newly activated or enhanced sex life. It's also important to note that changes in erection strength and function can be indicators of health problems not yet diagnosed. It is critically important that men receive an exam and evaluation from their primary care doctor or urologist before starting medications for erectile dysfunction, even if they can access them through unofficial channels.

Another interesting and often unexpected result is that when many men take these erection-restoring medications, it returns them to the vigor of younger days. (You might be thinking, *sounds great!*) My caution to men is this: just because your appendage is in youthful splendor, don't forget that the rest of your body is still seven decades in and parts may be out of warranty. How many men have come in with "sex trauma"—slipped discs, broken penis, strains, and sprains—because in the moment of rapture they lost track of their own body limitations? Many of these, most often orthopedic, limitations apply to women as well; hips that have become creaky with arthritis may respond in the moment, but when the euphoria passes, they suddenly seize up and become stiff and painful. When I mentioned a broken penis, I was not kidding. Penile fractures are a urologic emergency and delaying care will cause permanent damage to sexual function. If you are a man and, in the heat of the moment, you experience excruciating pain, an immediate loss of erection, and your penis looks like an eggplant, don't sit around and see if it gets better in a few days. Delayed care is not your friend. Another complication of erectile dysfunction medications is priapism, an erection that will not end. It is the cause of many jokes, but the truth of the matter is that this is also a urologic emergency and, left untreated, can result in permanent damage. One of my favorite urologists shared his experience with a gentleman who took a medication to assist his erection. Days later, when it had not gone down, he finally came into the office. By then the damage was done. He had developed fibrosis (permanent scarring) and his erections were never the same again.

I had a patient once come into the clinic and, with tears in her eyes, laughingly recount a "sex fail." In the heat of the moment, she rolled over on top of her partner, throwing a leg over him to be on top, when both of her hips went into full muscle spasm at the forced, and unprepared, flexibility requirement of this movement. She could neither get off nor stay up, consequently collapsing in an inglorious heap on her partner while yelling out loud in unexpected pain. It's safe to say the "moment" passed.

Since the goal of this book is to focus on sexually transmitted infections, I will defer to my geriatric specialty colleagues to write the book on some of these aging-related hurdles, and I will focus on the ones specific to infection. But it is an important consideration when quick-starting your sex life. Also important to reflect on in this section is the cultural and societal history for women and sexuality. Many women of the older generations think of their genitals as "dirty" and a "no fly" zone for self-touch. It is time to break those decades-old associations. The human body is beautiful. Sex is magical. No one should ever feel shame about how they look or how they feel when they are enjoying themselves sexually.

### Loss of Skin Elasticity

Both men and women suffer physical changes due to fading hormones, resulting in the tragic loss of skin elasticity. You might have noticed aging skin often gets wrinkly or paper-thin, and becomes less forgiving. A nip from a puppy creates a skin tear that takes weeks

to heal and bleeds for hours. The jagged edge from a briar while prun-
ing roses creates a tear that peels back the skin rather than just lodg-
ing itself. In my urgent care days, a shift did not pass me by when I was
not throwing a few stitches into a big skin flap from a minor injury in
an elderly patient. While mostly a nuisance and not dangerous by itself, this loss of elasticity plays out differently in the genital region,
particularly for women. Women, through the lack of estrogen, develop vaginal dryness and skin atrophy. Atrophy means that the
younger vaginal tissue, which is both flexible and ridged with rugae,
becomes flattened. For some women who go a very long time without
vaginal penetration, this can also create a "fusion" of the genital tissues, making it impenetrable. For all women experiencing age-related
loss of elasticity and moisture, friction with intercourse can create tiny
tears in the vaginal and vulvar tissue that create openings for infection and make them more prone to getting an infection from their
partner. Sometimes these changes impair sensation, and friction that
used to feel amazing suddenly burns or creates discomfort.

A dear friend shared a story with me. She and her new partner,
both in their mid-70s, decided to have a "go" at sex. She had not been
sexually active for almost two decades and recounted the story to me
as "funny later, but not at the time!"

"No matter how hard we tried," she said, "which included a mid-
night run to an all-night pharmacy to buy two different kinds of lubricant, he just couldn't get it in!"

She shared that it was not just painful for her but also incredibly
embarrassing. She went to her family doctor, who diagnosed her with
adhesions—essentially, the skin had "grown together." This was
treated with topical estrogen, and after a short time, resolved. The pa-
tience and understanding of her partner in the moment made the
experience bearable, but it is easy to imagine a scenario where it could
have been both physically and emotionally very distressing. How great
that this woman felt comfortable going right to her family doctor to

talk about, and resolve, the issue and that there was, truly, a happy ending!

Another challenge many women will experience with age is urinary incontinence and uterine and/or bladder prolapse, which means the connective tissues that used to hold everything firmly in place have relaxed and cause the bladder to empty when least expected. At times, with age and weakening of the supporting muscles, the bladder or uterus, or even both, can "fall down." They remain like this unless manually replaced with something called a "pessary" or with surgery. Many tales exist of "home remedies," such as pessaries created out of potatoes, made by people hesitant to go to their health care provider. With the loss of estrogen, many women will also leak urine during orgasm, which can significantly impair their ability to enjoy intimacy for fear of "having an accident." Organ prolapse and urinary incontinence can create embarrassment and discomfort and cause some women to avoid intimacy altogether. The good news is that many of these problems can be treated and cured by a talented urologist or gynecologist and should not be a cause for abstinence.

Women of all ages can experience urinary tract infections related to sex. It is often referred to as "honeymooners" syndrome, based on increased intercourse frequency of newlyweds and the resultant urinary tract infections that are not due to a sexually transmitted infection. The same can happen in older adults as well when they refresh sexual activity. Many of the above-mentioned aging changes can also contribute to increased bacteria moving into the urethra and creating a nidus of infection. But sometimes, particularly when a woman has not had infections in a long time, it can be a sign of a sexually transmitted infection. This is particularly concerning when urine cultures are negative for bacteria but symptoms recur.

One of my colleagues, a physician I have known since my own early doctor days, confided in me about a patient she once had. She reflected back with some remorse that she didn't push more aggressively for STD testing. She shares this memory:

> I took care of a couple in their early 70s. She had pretty advanced multiple sclerosis (MS) and was wheelchair-/bed-bound. He was a very active, social guy, with minimal health problems, who had remained active in the community. He was out and about a lot while she was home with a caregiver, but he always brought her in for regular appointments.
>
> She would periodically come in with rip-roaring urinary tract infections (UTIs), but that's not necessarily unusual with MS. With one of these, I did a bit more of a gynecologic exam and talked with her. Of course, her vaginal tissues were paper-thin/atrophic and appeared irritated. She somewhat reluctantly stated that her husband had had intercourse with her, that it was uncomfortable, but also that she did not object to this. In going back over her record, it appeared her times of the rip-roaring UTIs corresponded with times of intercourse.
>
> She insisted she did not wish me to say anything to her husband about this, and she made it clear that she consented and would continue to do so. She was fully competent and a very well-educated lady. All I could do was try to discuss some other forms of sexual activity that didn't involve vaginal penetration/urethral disruption, as well as increased lubrication.
>
> This went on for a couple years. She actually had fewer episodes of UTIs. She did tell me one time that she felt her husband was spending "a lot" of time away from the house with all his activities, and this bothered her. Unfortunately, her overall health sharply declined about that time, and she ended up passing away. Within a couple of months, the husband remarried a younger woman.

This has always bothered me somewhat through the years. I wondered if I should have been more forward in talking with the husband, even though the wife was clear that she did not desire that. Certainly, she consented to the sexual activity; I think she saw it as one way to hang on to his affection and care for her. Looking back, I also wonder if I should have looked more into STDs. Was he "running around" on her?

It can be difficult and uncomfortable to suggest to patients, especially those in long-term monogamous relationships, that they have symptoms of a sexually transmitted infection. It is especially challenging when the primary care physician cares for both partners in a marriage. Despite that discomfort, any woman with a sudden onset of recurring urinary tract infections that do not culture positive for a bacterium definitely needs testing for sexually transmitted infections.

So, what's a woman to do? Uncertainty about the risk associated with hormone replacement therapy has made these systemic treatments not possible for many women, but new research reassures us that topical use is safe for many women. Many women who cannot take oral hormone replacement can still benefit from locally applied topical estrogen that can bring aging tissue back toward near-youthful splendor. Using a lubricant for penetration can create more pleasurable friction. Just as erectile dysfunction can feel shameful to men, some women are embarrassed about their ability to show excitement with natural lubrication and may suffer discomfort rather than speak up. Like all things "intimate," it is critical to be able to share with your partner if you are having discomfort with sex. If that still sounds impossible to you, at the very least share your concerns with your primary care provider or gynecologist, as there are other daily-use suppositories that some women might use to create a more moist environment that can make sex more pleasurable. Not only will this enhance the physical experience, but it also creates protection against unwanted infections. For over-the-counter remedies, be sure to go to reliable resources to identify the best solution for you.

Thin skin and loss of elasticity create a risk of infection for men as well but in a different way. One of my colleagues shared a story of a patient in his mid-70s who decided to put himself on the market, and with the help of a dating app and an erection aid, he became quite sexually active. It was all fun and games until he came into the office with a wicked herpes outbreak. Due to not using condoms, his risk was increased because of those microscopic tears in the skin—tears you cannot see with the naked eye—that create openings for infection. It's important to be on the lookout because this gentleman declared that unprotected sex far outweighed the nuisance of these pesky ulcers, and he declined any other STD testing, putting him and his future sexual partners at risk not only for genital herpes but also for whatever else might be brewing.

## Weakening Immune Function

Another topic in the "biology of aging" for us to consider is that our immune response is not as strong as we age, making it harder for our systems to naturally fight infection. Infections that might have been transient or self-resolving when we were younger are more likely to persist and worsen with age. For instance, the decreased ability to fight off COVID-19 clearly showed that the population over 65 had much worse outcomes with infection. The same can be true of sexually transmitted infections in older adults. The vaccines that might create a robust immune response in a young person may simply not be that effective for older adults, which means that the vaccines for sexually transmitted infections like HPV are not made available to older adults. The Advisory Committee on Immunization Practice (ACIP) establishes standard, evidence-based guidelines for HPV vaccination and supports vaccination up to age 45 but not after because the vaccine is not FDA approved beyond that age.

Only you will know if you are physically able and interested enough to enjoy sex and intimacy with aging, but rest assured that sex is on the mind of many older adults. According to an article published on the AARP website, the neighborhoods where retirees have formed large communities have the steepest, most dramatic increase in STD rates: "[In] Arizona's Maricopa and Pima counties—home to large retirement communities just outside Phoenix—the percent[age] of reported cases of syphilis and chlamydia increased twice as fast as the national average from 2005 to 2009. Reported cases were up 87% among those fifty-five and older in those counties."

One of my good friends, Glady, recently shared how excited she was that her mid-70s mother had moved close by into a condo in a retirement community. It was a perfect scenario. Glady retained her space and avoided tension with an "in-law" in residence, and her mother, Ellen, preserved her space and didn't feel pressured or obligated to live under someone else's roof. They could support each other through illness or surgery. Her mom also got to restart with a ready-made community and was able to socialize, attend local events, and enjoy retirement on her own terms. The mother–daughter duo enjoyed weekly lunches together, and during one such lunch her mother regaled her with a story from her new home.

"I was at dinner with my mom and her friends the other night. They were the older ladies that mom hangs out with. They are all well into their 80s," Glady started. "So, a man walked by the table and Ellen harrumphed and said that he's one to avoid."

"Avoid? Why?" I asked her. Honestly, I had no idea what she was talking about.

"Well," Glady continued, "Apparently he is quite the player! Liz said that he has S-E-X with a lot of the ladies, and I should stay away from him."

"Is your mom sexually active?" I interrupted.

"No! Ewwwwwwwwww. No!"

"Well, if she is, I hope she's being careful."

Glady went back to her story as if I had not just suggested her mom might be enjoying a healthy and active sex life in her new retirement community.

"Anyway, one of my mom's friends is pretty deaf. So, she says, 'S-E-X at this age is like stuffing a marshmallow in a parking meter!' She said it loud enough for everyone to turn their heads and stare at us. My mother could've died! You should've seen how red their faces were." All the ladies had a good laugh.

The next time I saw Glady, I asked her how her mom's sex life was going and she just rolled her eyes and walked away. Whether she likes it or not, her mom very well may find a new love in the community.

## Iatrogenic Complications of Aging

Everything we have discussed so far in the "biology of STDs" has been inherent biology, but some of the changes are actually iatrogenic, meaning they are caused by the treatments themselves as we navigate chronic disease. Many older adults take chronic medications, and what's even more concerning is that many are simultaneously on multiple medications (what we call in medicine "polypharmacy") that can contribute to immune dysfunction, erectile dysfunction, dry skin and mucosa, and decreased sexual desire, among other things. Suffering from some of these means some people will choose to avoid intimacy, which puts their risk for a sexually transmitted infection quite low. Others will not and become more susceptible to infection. Add to this the fact that common treatments for STDs, which are not concerning for younger generations who are not on medications, can create dangerous drug interactions in patients with chronic illness who are on complex medicine regimens.

Health care providers must weigh the pros and cons of stopping one medicine to treat an infection versus taking a risk of drug interactions. The risk–benefit ratio is a foundation of medical training. In the past decade the patient has been brought into this conversation even more intentionally with "shared decision-making." It is very important that whoever treats you for any potential sexually transmitted infections is fully aware of your medical regimen in order to avoid a dangerous outcome and that they involve you as the key decision-maker in your care.

Devon had struggled with high blood pressure since early childhood, and it worsened until it became so severe that even with five medicines it was not controlled. In renal failure and on dialysis by his 40s, a condition further complicated by heart failure, he was close to giving up on life. But just a few months prior to coming in to see us at the STD clinic, he received a life-changing call: a kidney was available! What followed was a whirlwind of labs, imaging, and preoperative evaluations, all culminating in a new kidney and a renewed lease on life. By the time I saw him, he was smiling ear to ear.

He had come into the STD clinic for genital warts. He had a long-time partner who had been with him for decades. There was no promiscuity on his part or hers, but he had struggled with a bout of genital warts in his late adolescence. Since the transplant, they had begun to grow back with a vengeance. On examination, he had mounds of warts on his penis, peppering his scrotum, his perineum, and all around his anal area. They were marching like ants across his nether regions.

The immune-suppressing drugs that kept his body from rejecting the foreign kidney had reactivated what was an old and forgotten HPV infection. This was a great reminder of two things: (1) the nature of viral STDs is that they persist even if you cannot see them, and (2) the power of the immune system is mighty. Medications or conditions that weaken immunity create opportunities for infection.

## Treatments: Merry-Go-Round

One of the big challenges in health care with the advent of clinical studies and evidence-based medicine (which is overall a great thing) is that the recommendations change really frequently. One of the things this book is not going to do is spell out how each infection is treated specifically because, statistically speaking, it's going to change. The combination of drug resistance, new emerging drugs, existing drugs in the United Kingdom that don't have US approval, and a myriad of other factors mean the treatment world is constantly evolving. There is also a risk that Internet "doctors" (admit it, you've been there yourself!) try a gazillion over-the-counter and self-treatments for symptoms of infection before going in. There is a lot of risk to this in the sexual health arena. As you will learn in subsequent chapters, some infections seem like they go away but are not really gone. For a variety of reasons, including the fact that the treatment recommendations keep changing, I am going to steer away from specific treatments (curative and symptom relief) in this book and leave that to your primary care provider.

## The Biology of STDs

Humans are amazing biologic creatures, but so are viruses and bacteria. Take, for instance, gonorrhea. In my 20-plus years of treating STDs, I have seen no fewer than six different recommended antibiotic regimens, with a seventh just announced because that wily bacterium so rapidly develops drug resistance.

No sooner do we have a new regimen than we must change it to counter the bacteria's ability to resist the drug. The biology of microorganisms creates a whole layer of risk for successfully treating sexually transmitted infection. In 2018, the first completely drug-resistant strain of gonorrhea was identified in the United Kingdom, spurring a flurry of research and development for novel antibiotics. Recent episodes of fully drug-resistant gonorrhea have heightened fears of the development of full resistance across the United States as well (fig. 2.1). What do we do when we have nothing left with which to treat gonorrhea?

Among the STDs, we are watching more than gonorrhea develop drug resistance. Many infections are becoming resistant to treatments. One of the newest on the scene, *Mycoplasma genitalium* (which you will learn more about in chapter 4) developed resistance to multiple antibiotics almost immediately upon discovery. Many of the sexually transmitted viral infections, like hepatitis C and HIV (chapter 5), have an uncanny ability to develop drug resistance, forcing medicine to pivot and modify treatment regimens to continue to be able to suppress them.

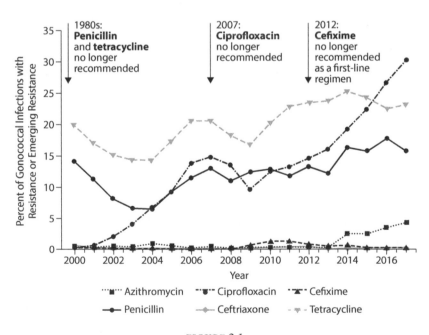

FIGURE 2.1.
Resistance of gonorrhea to antibiotic treatment. *Source:* cdc.gov

While the bacteria and viruses plague us with their ability to dodge modern medicine, we have come huge distances in our ability to diagnose these infections rapidly and accurately. With each infection in the following chapters, I will share the different tests that aid the diagnosis and identify which is most accurate.

## A History Lesson

I will close our second chapter together with one of my favorite trips into the past and the most dramatic historical STD diagnosis and treatment story I know. It is the story of syphilis.

The true origin of syphilis is heavily debated. Some say it was "discovered" by Christopher Columbus and brought back from the New World in the 1400s (the Columbian theory). Others claim that it goes back even further, to the 1200s, when there was a form of "leprosy" that was suspiciously similar to syphilis. Lastly, there is the "evolutionary theory," which suggests it dates back much, much further in time.

Syphilis was the cause of "the Pox" (not to be confused with smallpox or monkeypox) and spread rapidly in Europe in the late 1800s. Stories about historical figures like William Shakespeare, Abraham Lincoln, and Oscar Wilde reveal that throughout history, STDs have posed a risk for everyone, not just the marginalized and disenfranchised. In a scholarly article on the history of syphilis, the author states, "Great syphilitics of history are said to include Ivan the Terrible, Henry VIII, Toulouse Lautrec, Randolph Churchill and Al Capone."

Given the lack of diagnostic testing at the time, these stories are all based on descriptions of ailments, but it is an interesting "Who's Who." I confess that I am not even an amateur historian, so I will keep the history lesson brief, but we can learn a lot from syphilis, and true scholars have written many articles about the history of this clever sexually transmitted infection, which continues to be a prominent public health threat even today.

The early syphilis treatments were devastating. They included horrific tools like mercury steam boxes, where a person was placed in a sealed box and vaporized mercury was piped in, which had an equal probability of killing and curing. Mercury was the only potential treatment available until the discovery of Salvarsan in the 1900s and, finally, penicillin in 1943. Metal tools to inject mercury directly into the urethra of the penis were also used (and were purportedly discovered on Blackbeard's ship—arrrrgh, matey!). The use of mercury led to the public health saying, "Two minutes with Venus, two years with Mercury." These treatments, however, were preferable to the suffering and ultimate death from the infection and so were sought despite their often-dire consequences.

In chapter 4 you will learn all the secrets of syphilis, but to understand these images now, understand that syphilis presents in three stages as the disease progresses. By the time you reach the third stage, the infection erodes the cartilage, which then collapses. Because no definitive treatment was available and antibiotics were not even a glimmer in the eyes of physicians back then, many sufferers would progress to tertiary syphilis, creating a market for "artificial noses" to replace the ones that had been destroyed by the infection.

One of the most atrocious unethical studies in the history of medicine came much later, in the 1930s, with the Tuskegee Syphilis Study undertaken in Alabama by the US Public Health Service. This study created one of the many blights on medical history that has fostered a valid distrust of medicine and furthered health disparities. In this study, poor Black men, mostly sharecroppers, were enrolled to follow the natural course of syphilis to learn how the disease progressed without treatment. They were told the study would last six months and were offered free health care in exchange, but they were not told that "free health care" meant placebo treatment only. Even with the advent of penicillin in the 1940s, none of the men were treated, though free burial insurance was provided as a "benefit" of being in the study. Despite the initial projection of a short trial, this historically unethical syphilis trial continued for 40 years—resulting in the pain, suffering, and death of many trial subjects and the spread of syphilis to women and their unborn babies.

From the Pox of the 1400s to the socially unjust experimentations of yesterday, we have traveled tremendous distances in understanding and treating sexually transmitted infections over time, and our understanding of the aging process and ability to treat many of the symptoms of aging has never been better. We can diagnose infections early and easily, and tests are available to all older adults free or at generally low cost. With all the advancements in science and progress of researchers and physicians, one is left to ask: Why are STDs rising at such an alarming rate in the older population? What's driving the rise, and why aren't we in control of it?

## CHAPTER 3

# The Good, the Bad, and the Ugly

Sex indiscretions lead to depression,
No matter how you like it, condoms give the best protection.


LUIS WORKED ODD JOBS and cared for his aging parents, who were well into their 70s and lived in his home. He had never acknowledged his sexual orientation publicly or to his family privately, and he had no intention of letting them know before they passed away that he was gay. Living with his elderly parents strained his social life and made long-term relationships virtually impossible. Over the prior year, he had heard friends talking about dating apps to find casual, one-time partners, and he decided to try it. He didn't believe he would ever be able to experience a loving long-term relationship, but that didn't mean he couldn't let off some steam. It worked! Within months he had amazing sexual experiences with quite a few new partners and never had to worry about the awkwardness of hiding a relationship or being discovered. His family was deeply rooted in traditional Latino Catholicism, and he didn't think his parents could accept knowing that their son was gay. It would devastate them. Hiding his sexuality meant that he didn't have to worry about having awkward conversations or exposing himself to vulnerable feelings, certain that his parents could not accept this truth about him. It meant that he could preserve the relationship with his parents without the fear of judgment or abandonment while still being able to satisfy his own sexual needs and desires. But although this situation offered a solution to one problem, it presented many other dangerous complications in the long run.

Not long into his newfound sexual freedom, while he was running on the treadmill at the local gym, someone tapped him on the shoulder. He turned to see Tom, a hookup from the month before. Tom awkwardly explained that he was lucky to have tracked him down because he had been diagnosed with syphilis only days after their "date" and had not been able to reach him. He encouraged Luis to get tested since he had no idea which of them was the source of the infection.

Thankfully, Luis took Tom's advice and came to my clinic for testing right away. He got a shot of penicillin while waiting for his test results, and we did all the other recommended screening based on his risk factors. Amazingly, the syphilis test ended up being negative (though because very early infection can result in a "false negative" test, with his known contact he still needed treatment). Unfortunately, what we did not expect was that he would test positive for chlamydia in both his throat and rectum. He had no symptoms at all. Did he get those infections from Tom, or did he give them to Tom? What about all the people both he and Tom had been with since they were together who might now have an infection and not know it? How would he find Tom to warn him? The stress of this unexpected outcome of using technology to identify sexual partners was eye-opening. He realized how lucky he was to not be infected with HIV and committed to using condoms from then on.

In this chapter we are going to get up to speed on trends in the sexual health world as it relates to using technology for relationships, examine how sexual networks have changed, and learn about the all-important, and often not understood, world of extragenital infections.

## "Hookup" Dating Applications

The advent of social media and online dating applications has exploded sexual networks and created astonishing pathways for infections to spread across the world almost overnight. Casual hookups are not the only ones aided by this technology; long-lasting love can also be found online. According to eHarmony, 20% of current, committed relations begin online, and senior dating sites are on the rise. In a 2016 interview, cofounder of Coffee Meets Bagel, Dawoon Kang, told NBC News, "In 2014 and 2015 we saw 81 percent and 314 percent growth in registration among the 55–64 group." Those numbers have continued to grow since then. My guess is, yes, Grandma probably knows how to swipe right. Back in 2002, during my residency, I remember being at the gym, kickboxing on a Saturday morning with a fellow resident. In between chops and jabs she told me she had met someone online and they had gone out a few times. At that time, she felt that it was embarrassing for her to admit she had turned to technology to find a mate. In the early 2000s, dating apps rang of desperation, as opposed to today, when they have become the norm. I am glad to say that she and her partner have now been married almost 20 years and represent a relatively early success story of Internet love. Wow, how times have changed!

One of my son's friends came home from fall break freshman year of college to visit. We were enjoying a cup of coffee at the bar, and I was quizzing her about college life. She very casually mentioned meeting up with someone she had met on an app. *Oh no*, I thought, *here we go again!* Having treated so many STDs related to casual sexual hookups in her generation, I was genuinely worried about her health and safety. This was a great kid, and I wasn't sure she knew how risky that choice was.

"Whoa! You have to be careful finding partners that way! I am seeing some of my worst STDs from these hookup apps," I warned.

My son rolled his eyes and his friend blushed, saying, "No, like, to be a friend. It's really hard to meet people."

She was lonely and had not found her tribe at the huge university, and so she was using the app as a friend finder—with great success, I might add. This was incredibly eye-opening for me. Prior to this, my skepticism of the choice to use dating apps was high because I was seeing all of the bad outcomes in the form of unleashed sexually transmitted infections. This young coed opened my eyes to some of the intrinsic value of these tools.

There are numerous online reviews of these dating apps for those who have an interest in learning more. "There are plenty of other mature singles who are looking for anything from a casual hookup partner to a traveling companion or workout buddy," starts a Mashable blog from January 2021 that evaluates the top 10 Best Senior Dating Sites. Before you decide if online dating is your cup of tea, I think it is wise to break down some of the positives and negatives of using technology to find relationships.

## The Positives of Hookup Apps

The biggest positive of dating sites goes far beyond identifying a casual sex partner or even a long-lasting love. Finding company for dinner, a tennis date, a travel companion, or a mentor are all ways an online dating app might be used to change your life. They have been shown to provide a source to match young people not ready to come out with anonymous mentors who can assist in their journey. This is an amazing tool that was simply not an option in the past for so many people who identify as homosexual.

I think back to one of my dear friends in medical school who was failing out of school. I went to his apartment one night to talk and see if I could offer assistance with his studies. He confessed, ashamed and in tears, that he was gay. He had tried hard not to be. His parents did not understand or approve and had forced him to go through conversion therapy—to no avail, naturally. He was navigating all that, essentially alone, while trying to learn how to be a doctor. It was just too much. If he'd had the benefit of convenient, long-distance mentors to offer support at his fingertips, from the comfort of his home, in between cramming for endless exams, that year of his life would have looked very different. It is one of the many ways I have come to appreciate some of the very strong positive impacts of using technology to develop relationships and provide needed support from incredibly broad geography and diversity.

A close family friend of mine recently spent a few months in Florida after his wife was admitted to a skilled nursing facility for her dementia. It had been a tumultuous decade of watching his love of over 50 years wrestle with mind-shattering nightmares, personality changes, and the slow and gradual loss of self. Because of the COVID-19 pandemic, which resulted in massive restrictions on hospitals and nursing homes, he was not allowed to visit her in the new facility where he had intended to spend time each day. He was bereft. His children encouraged him to go back to the community they had lived in for several years to get some sun and take care of himself until he was able to visit his wife in person, and he finally agreed. Curious to know how pandemic life was affecting senior living communities, I asked him to find out the lay of the land down there in the Florida retirement world, where the urban legends are pretty darn impressive. (Urban legends are stories passed along based on word-of-mouth that are often exaggerated or blown out of proportion.) Stories about great "sex-capades" in retirement communities are numerous, like the description of The Villages as the "Disneyland for seniors" in an article in *Lake & Sumter Style*, which goes on to mention that the reputation is well deserved.

The articles states, "A few Villages residents were arrested for having sex in golf carts, on town squares, and even on a utility box in recent years."

My friend was a shy man who was not willing to frequent bars and nightclubs or tie loofahs to his golf cart (presumably to indicate sexual preferences), but he was willing to develop a profile and go on a dating app to do some "recon" and look for platonic companionship. He was lonely, heartbroken, and at sea by himself, and when I asked for help doing senior research, I honestly hoped this would give him, at worst, a distraction and, at best, a new friend. He called me a few weeks later with an update.

"Shannon, I did what you asked. I got an account, and I have talked to a few people." He paused. I could hear him thinking. "I just don't know how to do this. I mean, my heart is with my wife. You go 50 years with someone and then suddenly there is no one to share a meal with, to reflect on the sunset with. . . . It feels disloyal to be doing this."

We talked for a while that Saturday morning, as I sat by the fire watching the snow come down outside and he basked in the southern sun on his balmy porch with his dog. While it was not the right time for him to meet people, even in the interest of my research, he said that he saw some real value in how these apps can help people connect. He shared some of his findings. Many women were looking for intimacy, plain and simple. Others were looking for life mates and were not interested in casual relationships; instead, they wanted to find "the one" to spend their sunset years with. Others were looking for companionship without sex. The options were seemingly endless. Apps like Our Time, Silver Seniors, and Match are helping to bring people together in a powerful way that is truly amazing.

Other apps that can have positive results are some of the confidential "disclosure" apps where someone can alert another person that they tested positive for an STD without having to say who they are. This has the potential to ultimately increase partner treatment without having to identify themselves. Many offer at-home testing and options for virtual treatment when a person tests positive. The convenience brought about by technology continues to impress and amaze!

*Alexa's Story*

Several years after Alexa's husband died, her daughter helped her set up a profile on eHarmony. She had seen how successful her daughter's dating life had been. Her daughter's match resulted in a marriage. However, Alexa was looking for a companion, not to marry; just date.

She was pleasantly surprised with the results. Before he passed, Alexa's husband had been ill for years and his illness took their fabulous sex life away. She loved him so much that it just didn't matter. She thought sex was over for her. Not so! She met a man that she connected with both physically and emotionally. They are still together after three years.

"Sex is great with the help of modern medicine. Who knew I would be loving the sex??!?" wrote Alexa, now aged 71.

## The Negatives of Hookup Apps

Unfortunately, like Newton's law of motion, which states that for every action there is an equal and opposite reaction, dating apps bring a host of negatives to balance out the positives. A mentor helping a young man find support through his journey toward acknowledging and accepting his homosexuality might actually be a sexual predator. That college student sitting alone in her cramped dorm room looking for a friend may spend all her time in solitude, scrolling through dating apps, glued to her device. That sweet old man looking for love that you happened to swipe right on—what if he smothered his wife with a pillow? (Okay, okay, I will admit that's an extreme example, but you get my point.) Sexual predators are a known hazard of these anonymous programs, where you can cut and paste a picture of anyone and invent a fictional existence to meet your every need. There are even television shows that explore this phenomenon called "catfishing," and it happens much more often than one might expect.

Catfishing is not, as it turns out, about dropping a real hook in the water, but metaphorically it is pretty close. This is when someone creates a completely false persona to lure people into their life. They keep up this act to reach some desired purpose. Perhaps they are cruel and delight in manipulating others. Perhaps they are scammers or financial predators. Perhaps they are truly unhappy with who they really are and this is a harmless attempt to reinvent themselves. A blog article on Phys.org states that loneliness was mentioned by 41% of respondents as the reason for their catfishing.

But whatever the motivation, the outcome is never good.

Online dating is clearly not for everyone. In a *Newsweek* article from February 28, 2021, Jon Berger, author of the book *Make Your Move*, writes, "According to Pew Research, 55% of women believe dating is harder today than it was 10 years ago. Two troubling reasons why: 57% of women report experiencing harassment on dating apps, and 19% say they've even been threatened with physical violence."

Perhaps more notable is what is described as "problem use" (an addiction of sorts) that can consume and control a user's life. The majority of people who use dating apps actually use several simultaneously since they are often marketed to different audiences—a constant pinging of potential partner messages, app-generated partner suggestions, and maintaining your profile can become incredibly time-intensive (and then you have to leave time for the actual "dates"). Every few months a new research study emerges about problem use—in essence, an inability to curb or stop use such that it dominates one's life. It can materialize in the same way as other addictions, like gambling, overeating, drinking, and drugs. This addiction to social media and particularly dating sites is problematic for teens and adults alike.

Problem use of hookup apps can be a recipe for potential disaster, especially if you meet certain criteria: the two factors most closely associated with developing problem use are—ironically—loneliness and social anxiety. Researchers from Ohio State University published a study in 2020 on this issue and discovered that there is a statistically significant risk of problem use for individuals with these features. They stated, "Although these emerging technologies offer social benefits, certain individuals become overly dependent on such applications and suffer from negative outcomes."

Just as Internet-based pornography addiction is a burgeoning threat among very young teens, dating apps can trigger similar compulsive behaviors that can prove not only disruptive but dangerous for lonely, older adults.

One of my colleagues in medicine sat on a national commission with me. We would see each other two or three times a year at these centralized meetings. She was single and dated a great deal. She was comfortable with casual dating and very brief hookups. Her travels always included meeting up with someone new on one of her apps while at these conferences. It consumed her. Rather than paying attention to the board agenda, I would find her swiping and pausing, swiping and pausing. It distracted from her meaningfully engaging as a board member, and it opened her life up to significant risks in the form of sexually transmitted infections.

The website of Athena Health states, "Between 2014 and 2017, diagnosis rates for herpes simplex, gonorrhea, syphilis, chlamydia, hepatitis B, and trichomoniasis rose 23% in patients over the age of sixty." Yesterday's "playing the field" is a very different game today because of the exponential rise in sexually transmitted infections in the past decade. According to the CDC, "approximately one in five people in the U.S. had an STI on any given day in 2018, and STIs acquired that year will cost the American healthcare system nearly $16 billion in healthcare costs alone."

How does technology contribute to this situation? One of the most serious and potentially deadly unintended consequences of social media is a combination of the spread of asymptomatic infections and the anonymity of dating apps, which makes it difficult to reliably track partners when infections are discovered. Anecdotally, I would estimate that over half of the patients I care for in the STD clinic have used, or are actively using, hookup apps to find partners. Some use them regularly and some only occasionally, but it is a very common theme. If someone is using an alias because they are truly looking for a "one-time" hookup, it can be impossible to track them down to alert them that they have spread, or been exposed to, a sexually transmitted infection. There is also the risk of people intentionally spreading infections and making it impossible for public health officials to track them down and hold them accountable for this potentially deadly behavior. Dating apps are the inspiration for one of my STD limericks, which I call "Bad Strategy Blues," composed after a particularly bad day with a series of patients in the STD clinic who seemed genuinely surprised that they had succumbed to infections after numerous anonymous, unprotected hookups:

> "Bad Strategy Blues"
> I confess this Friday, I'm weary.
> I mean, really, why would you be teary?
> Eight new connections,
> Not a one with protection?
> Not a very strategic game theory!

Finally, and less likely to be an issue for the aged but certainly a concern for your kids and grandkids, dating apps provide a veritable playground of opportunity for sexual predators. There are worse online dating situations than catfishing. There are those who are engaging in truly predatory behavior. One of my colleagues had a young teen daughter who would secretly take pictures of herself in varying states of undress, post them, and get (predictably) overwhelmingly positive praise from the mystery men and women who saw them. She was just 13 years old. When her parents discovered what she was doing, they found numerous message exchanges that suggested the person writing to their child was not also a 13-year-old. That kind of positive reinforcement when you are an insecure middle schooler is hard to resist. Imagine if one of those connections was local and suggested an innocent "meet up" after school—what might follow? The risk of sex trafficking, a coercive relationship, an assault, or even murder is real.

An article in *ProPublica* in 2020, "Tinder Lets Known Sex Offenders Use the App. It's Not the Only One," tells the tragic story of Carole, a Harvard-educated entertainment executive. According to the article, Match connected her with a six-time convicted rapist who, she reported, had raped her on their second date.

An analysis of sexual assault victims who had used dating sites cited by CJI (Columbia Journalism Investigations) found that "in 10% of the incidents, dating platforms matched their users with someone who had been accused or convicted of sexual assault at least once."

## Technology: The Bottom Line

Let's say for our purposes that you personally have no intention of getting hooked on hookup apps and are not even sure you will ever use one. Perhaps you live in a retirement community where you are surrounded by potential partners all the time and are fully COVID vaccinated and unconcerned about the pandemic. Or perhaps by the time you're reading this, the pandemic is a thing of the past. Perhaps you plan on serial monogamy and are not interested in casual partners. Or maybe you are clear that you are interested in a partner, accompanied by some intimacy, but sex is not on the menu. Why should you worry about other people using technology to meet their sexual needs?

The biggest risk is asymptomatic infections. This refers to someone, like our friend Luis from earlier, who has an active and contagious infection (in his case, chlamydia in his bottom and throat) but does not have any physical indications. Asymptomatic spread is one of the driving reasons why the CDC has published such clear criteria for routine STD screening in its STI Guidelines. In chapter 8 we will explore what screening you might need based on these guidelines. Screening for asymptomatic infections is so important that it is why most insurance plans measure health care providers on "quality of care" based on whether all young women of reproductive age have a chlamydia test every year until they are 24 regardless of symptoms. The National Committee on Quality Assurance justifies this important quality metric because "75% of chlamydia infections in women and 95% of infections in men are asymptomatic."

In 2019, guess what percentage of women got the recommended screening in the United States based on their data? Half! The rates ranged from 47% to 58% depending on the type of plan, with Medicaid beneficiaries receiving the highest percentage.

Asymptomatic chlamydia and gonorrhea are also why every baby born in the United States today gets erythromycin ointment in their eyes upon birth—to treat potentially asymptomatic chlamydia infection in the mom, which could have been passed to the newborn's eyes during birth, causing permanent blindness.

The CDC's screening guidelines focus on the young because while sexually active young adults in the US make up only one-quarter of the sexually active population, they contract over one half of all STDs. The guidelines also focus on high-risk people—men who have sex with men, men and women using IV drugs, men and women who have multiple partners—but they do not spend much time or energy on the older population. The result is many seniors who are enjoying active sex lives but not benefiting from timely screening and diagnosis. From an "absolute volume" perspective, seniors have been a relatively small proportion of the total infections compared to adolescents and young adults, but the growth and trajectory of infections in this demographic is a cause for concern.

Asymptomatic sexually transmitted infections come in all shapes and sizes and infect a whole variety of body parts. It is estimated that one in five adults walking around has genital herpes; only about 10% of them know they have the infection because the rest have either no symptoms at all or such mild and infrequent symptoms that they don't realize there is a problem. One in three women who did not receive the HPV vaccine will be infected with HPV with their sexual debut and have no idea they have been infected. HPV is the virus that causes genital warts and a variety of cancers. In chapter 6 you will learn a great deal about the surge in cancers caused by this sexually transmitted infection.

## What Are Sexual Networks?

Remember Luis, whom I introduced you to at the top of the chapter? He was my patient who found out he was exposed to syphilis while running on a treadmill at the local Y and ended up with rectal and pharyngeal chlamydia. You will recall he had no symptoms at all. Asymptomatic sexually transmitted infections are incredibly common, and they spread like wildfire in sexual networks. Sexual networks were complicated enough before partners could easily be identified with a swipe on a smartphone. The inception of dating apps has connected individuals from across the globe in an unorthodox way, making the world feel a little smaller while STD rates rise precipitously.

It's really important to understand the concept of sexual networks. Let's take our friend Luis and set up an example of what a sexual network might look like. Maybe Luis was only hooking up with this one guy (let's call him Romeo for my literary-themed example). Since Romeo, as you will see, had other partners (who also had other partners), in essence, Luis was sharing body fluids much more broadly (fig. 3.1). This visual (apologies to the Bard for the poetic license I am employing) gives you an idea of the reality of what one hookup actually means for germ warfare. Luis had a great night out with Romeo, not realizing that Romeo had spent the day before in bed with Tybalt. Of course, Tybalt was hooking up with Benvolio (who was having a fling with Friar Tuck) and would occasionally hook up with Paris, who had four female partners. What felt like one partner on one occasion to Luis was really a whole cast of characters spreading infection unknowingly.

There is a great exercise I sometimes do with teen audiences when I am explaining the sexual network concept. You hand out a bunch of different kinds of cookies (I prefer Girl Scout cookies myself) and instruct the kids to hold the cookies and *not* to eat them. There is usually an astonishing amount of grumbling because everyone loves Girl Scout cookies. You have them feel them all over for the texture, bring them to their nose to smell them, inhaling deeply, and become

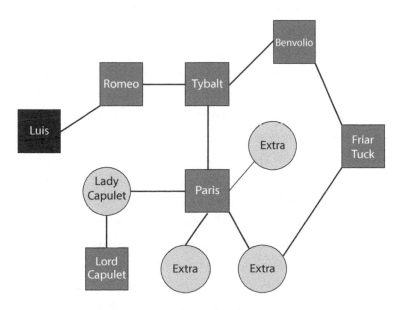

FIGURE 3.1.
Possible *Romeo and Juliet* hookups.

acquainted with the delightful dessert in their hands. Then you say, everyone with Thin Mints, trade them with people who have Caramel deLites. People with Caramel deLites, trade them for Peanut Butter Patties. You repeat the process of feeling them all over and smelling them. You do a few more trades. By now the cookies are *well* handled. You ask them, who wants to eat their cookies now? Every now and then you will find an eighth-grade boy who still wants to eat the cookie, but most kids are totally grossed out at this point. This is what sexual networks are like. The cookie still feels and smells the same, but it is most likely covered in germs!

## Men on the Down Low

You might notice in figure 3.1 that while Paris, a male who is publicly heterosexual, had four female partners, he also had a male partner. For this example, let's assume that Paris did not tell any of his female partners he occasionally dallied with men. Clearly, based on the diagram he is mostly heterosexual with four female partners, but it is the one male partner that significantly increases his risk for an infection (which in turn increases the risk for all of the women he is with).

The risk of sexually transmitted infections is higher in men who have sex with men. This phenomenon, known colloquially as "Men on the Down Low," has been around for all of history, but in the past decade it has been increasingly implicated in the spread of dangerous infections. Men on the Down Low are publicly heterosexual and have one or more female partners. Many of them are in committed relationships or monogamous marriages—except when they are not. These men have secretive sexual encounters with other men. They do not identify as homosexual or bisexual, and they do not share their occasional indiscretions with their partner(s). This phenomenon has contributed to the resurgence of congenital syphilis, an infection in pregnant moms that causes the unborn baby to die in the uterus or to be born infected with syphilis, which comes with significant consequences. In chapter 4 we will spend more time going into detail on the implications of syphilis infections.

## Extragenital Infections

Asymptomatic infections, Men on the Down Low, expanded sexual networks—what else could possibly go wrong? Extragenital infections: sexually transmitted infections outside of the vagina and penis. Yep, you heard it here first. Trust me, this is not like the "extra credit" you always wanted in school. Like our friend Luis, who had chlamydia in his rectum and throat, extragenital infections caused by bacteria and viruses are a burgeoning problem.

A 72-year-old man recently came into the clinic with a "funny spot" on his penis. He shared that he was happily married, for the most part, but that they had not been sexually active in many years. Every few years it would get to him and he would do something about it. He denied ever paying for sex but said he had recently been to a "massage parlor" and part of the service was oral sex. "I know it isn't a venereal disease," he said sincerely, "because we didn't have sex!" It never occurred to him that he could develop syphilis from oral sex.

Some extragenital infections are merely a nuisance, like a random genital wart (caused by HPV) that infects the mouth and tongue. Other times a different subtype of the same HPV virus can cause cancer. Rising rates of head and neck cancers in middle-aged adults implicate the HPV virus as the cause. Michael Douglas, Marcia Cross, and Farrah Fawcett were or still are advocates for HPV cancer awareness following their diagnoses.

Several recent studies have implicated saliva as a route for gonorrhea transmission—that's right, kissing can lead to gonorrhea! You might be asking yourself, is nothing safe? Eye infections have become problematic for teens and adults as well. We had three chlamydia diagnoses in eyes in the clinic last month! For the record, eye STDs are not from eye sex. I do a lot of STD talks to teens and young adults, and whenever I flash up a picture of a red, oozing eye with "gonorrhea" next to it, they collectively exclaim in horror. When I reassure them that it is *not* from eye sex, they look so relieved! Rather, I tell them that it's from touching infected body fluids—your own or your partner's—and then touching your eyes. Another sexually transmitted infection to assault the eye is syphilis. This sparked a CDC Special Provider Alert in 2016 warning health care providers to be vigilant for syphilis presenting with ocular (eye) symptoms.

Increasingly, public health is changing guidelines to reflect the rise in infections that occur outside of the penis and vagina. Many a throat and rectum are harboring infection that the "host" is totally unaware of. In the recent National Survey of Family Growth, which surveys men and women across the country about family, marriage, contraception, and other topics, we can see that the prevalence of men and women who engage in oral and/or anal sex continues to escalate in all age groups (fig. 3.2). These trends have persisted over the past decade, and a study released in 2018 reveals that 37% of the older adults surveyed had participated in oral sex in the prior year.

With 75% of both male and female adults engaging in oral sex and over 10% engaging in anal sex, the oral and anal mucosa have become the next frontier for sexually transmitted infections. We are learning that screening all areas of sexual exposure is critical to identify asymptomatic infections that might be a cause of the astonishing rates of sexually transmitted infections in this country.

### Virginity Pledges

I can't resist sharing a story about the movement in the late 1990s where teenagers and young adults made Virginity Pledges that inevitably failed in many ways for a variety of reasons. These pledges were commitments that were made, usually within a faith group, pledging that they would not have sexual intercourse until they were married. A review by the Guttmacher Institute in 2008 determined that "after

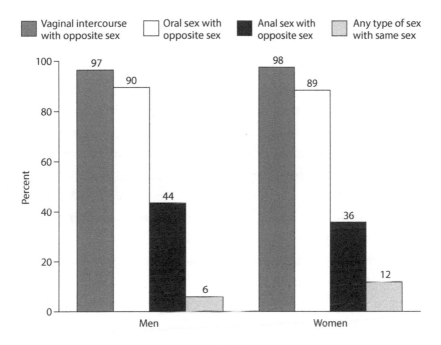

**FIGURE 3.2.**
Sexual behavior in lifetime among men and women aged 25 to 44 years in the United States from 2006 to 2008.
*Source*: cdc.gov

five years, more than half of both pledgers and nonpledgers had engaged in sexual activity, and the two groups had similar rates of sexually transmitted infections (STIs). Pledgers, however, were less likely to use contraceptives or to use them consistently."

The folly of any sort of abstinence approach to curbing the spread of STDs is flawed. Most humans are sexual creatures. Making sex shameful leads people to hide sexual activity to the point of avoiding taking measures for self-protection. Sadly, but not necessarily surprisingly, adolescents who took these pledges had higher rates of STDs and unintended pregnancy, and anal sex became a route to "preserving virginity." We can learn from these lessons and be sure to apply them with our friends, parents, or coworkers by making their sex lives a shame-free safe place for dialogue.

## It's Not Always Black and White

Martha, a recently retired executive, came to my office between regularly scheduled appointments with concerns of vaginal discharge.
She was married, monogamous, and did not think her husband had
been with anyone else. She only had receptive vaginal intercourse
(meaning a penis when in her vagina but not her mouth or rectum) but
acknowledged that they enjoyed a vigorous sex life. She vehemently
denied any extramarital relations herself. Her husband had retired a
couple years prior, and I saw a shadow of concern pass over her face
as she thought of his newfound free time.

On pelvic exam, her mucosa (the tissue of the vagina) was red and
inflamed, and her cervix had little red dots (broken blood vessels
called petechiae) and a lot of bubbly white discharge. This combination is highly suspicious of trichomonas. I took a sample on a long cot-
ton swab and looked at it under the microscope (this test is called a
"wet prep"). This showed organisms suspicious for trichomonads, but
it did not meet full diagnostic criteria of trichomonas because the organisms were dead, not wiggling around the slide (more on this in the
next chapter). A rapid trichomonas test in the office was positive.
Making the diagnosis of an STD in a happily married, presumably
monogamous couple is usually devastating, and it is always disruptive.
(In chapter 4 you will learn a great deal more about trichomonas, but
it is almost always and certainly a sexually transmitted infection.) I
recommended that she go home and have a very frank conversation
with her husband, and that he should get treated as well. Sending that
delightful 67-year-old woman home to have a very uncomfortable conversation was incredibly difficult. Ultimately, her husband denied
any possible risks and absolutely denied having any symptoms of
infection; the uncomfortable period in their marriage passed without a clear explanation for the uninvited guest.

This story begs the age-old question: Can you get an STD from a
toilet seat? As I tell my students in STD talks, it is exceptionally un-

likely. It is statistically improbable, like lightning-strike material. It would take such timing, such consecutive acrobatic-like seating precision, such an alignment of the stars, for this to occur that the alternative (someone brought it to a relationship) is exceedingly more likely. We know that viruses and bacteria can be shared on sex toys (more on sex toy hygiene later), which makes sense because it's a much more intimate experience and often involves fresh, hot body fluids in an immediate exchange and the toy is often inserted, providing ample opportunity to come into contact with and infect mucosa. However, the same viruses on a dry, solid surface simply don't remain infectious for long at all. Perhaps the hardiest of the buggers is trichomonas, which is reputed to enjoy a longer lifespan in moist environments such as loofah sponges.

The moral of these stories is this: There's a lot going on out there! When you become intimate or have sex with a new partner, be mindful. Statistically speaking, and especially if you met your partner on a hookup app, your partner is bringing you the risk of asymptomatic and/or extragenital infections. When you engage in new intimate relationships, even if they do not lead to sexual intercourse, many will lead to an exchange of body fluids, so you should always take the time to communicate with your health care provider about your sexual history and get screening tests on a reasonable and regular basis (more on this in chapter 8). In a perfect world, you would never enter into a new relationship without both of you (or all of you, depending on however many partners you engage with) getting tested in all the recently exposed body parts before you proceed so that everyone comes to bed with a clean slate.

## CHAPTER 4

# Treatable, Curable STDs

Bodies, we're just a cafeteria,
A cesspool of germs, viruses, and bacteria

MIKE, A MIDDLE-AGED BUSINESSMAN, came into the urgent care with a red, swollen, hot knee that he could barely bend. He described knee pain, fevers, and body aches that had started the day before. He had begun playing racquetball more in the few months prior and wondered if he had overexerted his knee. He was otherwise healthy, but he did have high blood pressure and cholesterol.

When I examined him in the office, I found that he had a low-grade fever. I explained the differential diagnosis to him, which included gout, monoarticular arthritis, or infection. He had never been diagnosed with or exhibited any symptoms of gout, never had problems with arthritis, and denied any recent cuts on his skin that would serve as openings for an infection to travel. He looked sick and his knee looked bad. Without any recent injury or a history of MRSA (methicillin-resistant *Staphylococcus aureus*, a bacterium that can cause big abscesses to form fairly quickly), and no reasonable medical history to give a clue to his diagnosis, I dug a little deeper.

"Any chance you have had a new sex partner recently?"

His eyes got very wide. He swallowed nervously and paused with his eyes downcast.

"Yes, last week, someone I met on a work trip. Why?"

"It's not terribly common," I explained, "but it is possible to get a sexually transmitted infection that can set up an infection in a joint.

Whenever we see a joint like yours, with this degree of infection, it usually needs the immediate attention of an orthopedic surgeon. I imagine he will need to take you to the operating room and clean your joint out under general anesthesia. At the very least you need IV antibiotics."

"Doc, I just got home. Can't you just put me on a medicine for a day or two and we just see how it does?" he pleaded.

"I'm sorry," I said. "The risk to your joint is permanent damage if we don't get the infection cleared out as soon as possible. Let me just send you over to the ER. I will call ortho and they will see you in the ER, and maybe they will be comfortable with a less aggressive plan," I suggested, though I knew there was no way he would not have a night in the hospital. Sometimes a little hope is the best medicine.

I promptly called the on-call orthopedic surgeon, who met him in the emergency room and took him to the OR to wash out his knee—which was filled with the pus of an infection with gonorrhea. The good news was that his infection was curable and treatable. The bad news? He had some explaining to do.

This is the "good news" chapter where I will tell you about the many wee beasties that might be a temporary nuisance but, if diagnosed in a timely fashion, can be vanquished almost overnight with modern medicine. Some require shots and some necessitate pills, some intravenous antibiotics, but all can ultimately be treated and cured. (There are also STDs that do not have outcomes quite as positive. We'll explore those shortly.)

Are you wondering what a wee beastie is? Did you know that when Dutch scientist Anton van Leeuwenhoek discovered some of the first moving organisms under a microscope in the seventeenth century, he called them "cavorting wee beasties"? When I learned this in sixth grade (it was the early 1980s), I was so excited that I promptly wrote a letter to the Kellogg Company (on our old-school typewriter) and suggested they name a breakfast cereal "Wee-beasties!" It did not occur to me that people might not be interested in eating viruses and bacteria for breakfast. I was sure I had a winning idea! It gets even worse. According to *Yale Medicine* magazine writer Ashley Taylor, the organisms van Leeuwenhoek was actually looking at and describing were in his own semen.

> "Preach it!"
> I preach condoms, but still they don't buy it!
> They stare blankly, respectfully quiet.
> With the sex drive of rabbits
> They need good sex habits—
> Our teens need a safer sex diet!

Three of the common bacterial infections (chlamydia, gonorrhea, and syphilis) are so contagious they are "reportable" to the Centers for Disease Control and Prevention. (This is the concept I introduced in chapter 3.) This means that when your health care provider diagnoses one of these infections, both the lab and the health care provider will complete a notification to the local health department. Each state manages reportable diseases differently based on their state public health statutes. For instance, in North Carolina, because of the volume of cases, only syphilis (of these three) is actively managed by state disease control specialists and tracked down with aggressive measures, such as repeated phone calls, home visits, and even court orders in extreme cases. The disease control nurses at local health departments review all reported diseases and verify that the diagnosing health care provider treated the infection correctly (which unfortunately does not always happen). The many changing treatment regimens present a challenge to health care practitioners, and sometimes going by memory rather than looking to see if guidelines have changed can result in inadequate treatments. At the local health department where I volunteer, gonorrhea is the most incompletely and incorrectly treated infection that we come across.

Sometimes a health care provider can treat the partner of their patient with a reportable STD without seeing the partner or having a health care provider–patient relationship with them. This is called expedited partner therapy (EPT). The ability to provide EPT varies by state. Where I am based in North Carolina, the only infections you can practically treat this way are chlamydia and gonorrhea. This means if I diagnose my patient with chlamydia, I can write a prescription for their partner to get treated without them having to pay for an office visit. If I stock the medication in my clinic, I can even dispense the medication for the partner to take. This increases the chance that both partners will be treated appropriately and in a timely fashion. If not, you run the risk of reinfection as the one who remains infected will likely infect the partner again, thus creating an STD cycle. Partner A gets treated and waits a week to resume condomless sex. Partner B gets treated but not until 10 days later, so effectively reinfects A before B is treated. And the infection persists! But there are risks to EPT for the health care provider: What if I treat Partner B and they are deathly allergic to the antibiotic, and I did not know that? Or what if it causes a drug–drug interaction that creates a devastating outcome? Some health care providers are not comfortable with expedited partner therapy for these reasons, and while it is an option in some states, it is never compulsory.

### Chlamydia: It's Not a Flower, Don't Wear It to Prom

Chlamydia is the most common of all the bacterial STDs. I've touched on it briefly, but it's time to delve in deeper. There is a great poster I saw back in the '90s with a cute teenage couple in prom attire and a caption that read: Chlamydia, it's not a flower. Don't wear it to the prom. Chlamydia is abundant and could even be described as ubiquitous in our young adult and adolescent female populations. Over the past decade, it has been creeping into the beds of the older population as well. Not a day goes by in the STD clinic without a diagnosis of chlamydia, and it is a muse for my limericks.

> "Looks Aren't Everything"
> Dear Chlamydia, your timing's not great,
> But it sure was a fabulous date!
> The fella looked clean
> (if you know what I mean)
> Perhaps PID's just a matter of fate.

Chlamydia is challenging because so many people are walking around with asymptomatic infections, so they pass it along unwittingly. Chlamydia is also happy to infect any mucosa it meets: the eyes, rectum, throat, vagina, and urethra are all fair game. It is also the cause of an infection that can develop around the liver and following infection, particularly in men, it can trigger a reactive arthritis that can last for weeks, months, or years following treatment. Most notably, chlamydia is incredibly common in young women. The often-asymptomatic infection wreaks havoc on the tiny tubes that carry eggs to be fertilized and creates scars and blockages that prevent pregnancy. It is also often the culprit for PID (pelvic inflammatory disease), which sometimes requires hospitalization and surgery. Infertility and chronic pelvic pain caused by chlamydia can be permanent and irreversible conditions.

Aside from the emotional toil of infertility, chlamydia is a tremendous medical expense in the United States—the most expensive STD according to a study published in 2013 in *Sexually Transmitted Diseases*. The study looked at the cost of infections in the prior decade and estimated a cost of as much as $775 million a year for chlamydia—and that was over a decade ago, so you can imagine with inflation what these numbers are now. Most people diagnosed with a chlamydia infection should return for a "test of reinfection" three months or so following treatment because often the partner is not treated simultaneously, and a reinfection follows that is asymptomatic but still causes complications. If there is concern about adherence to the regimen, persistent symptoms, or inability to complete the regimen, a "test of cure" is recommended in four weeks for select individuals.

How might you know if you have chlamydia? As I have mentioned before, many of you simply won't know. You will harbor the bacteria and share it with partners and not find out until you get a call from the health department or a kind partner. This is a perfect example of why screening is so important, because proper regular screening will keep you informed about your sexual health.

Some people with chlamydia do have symptoms. Women may have vaginal irritation or discomfort with penetration, and sometimes they experience spotting of blood after sex. This is more common in young women—any vaginal bleeding in a postmenopausal woman should prompt immediate evaluation by her health care provider. Postmenopausal bleeding may indicate something minor, like a polyp, or it can be a warning sign of cancer. Some women will notice an increase in discharge that is usually slightly discolored or will have crusting on their underwear that is new. Men's symptoms may include redness at the tip of their penis from the urethra being inflamed, a slight burning with urination that can be intermittent or persistent, or clear to white discharge, which can also show up subtly or as crusting on underwear. In my experience, men are so used to fluids coming out of their penises that they are rarely aware of subtle discharge. Numerous are the times when I have asked a man if he was having discharge and received a negative response, but when I examined them, it was very clearly there.

Treating chlamydia historically was very easy and gratifying because it was a one-time dose of antibiotics for some, or a week course for others, depending on a clinician's judgment about how likely it is that a patient will be able to reliably complete a week of medicine. Right there in the office, I can hand the pills and a cup of water to a patient and feel confident the bacterial infection is treated once they swallow them! If the partner(s) are treated at the same time, and everyone stays away from each other for a week, then the infection is cured. Unfortunately, because of myriad reasons including anonymous contacts, hesitancy to contact partners with bad news, an overwhelming volume of infections that the health departments cannot possibly manage, and inconsistent following of directions, chlamydia infection often returns or persists. Drug resistance is a concern but not a problem just yet, although the CDC changed the guidelines in 2021 to prefer a week's supply of medicine over a one-time dose. Additionally, there are numerous alternative treatment options using different antibiotics if a person is allergic to the recommended treatment (table 4.1).

TABLE 4.1. Basics of chlamydia

| | |
|---|---|
| Cause of Infection | *Chlamydia trachomatis, C. trachomatis* |
| Common Names | Chlamydia, CT, NGU |
| Type of Infection | Bacterial |
| Symptoms? | Variable, many asymptomatic |
| Duration of Infection | Weeks to years |
| What It Can Infect | Urethra, vagina, cervix, fallopian tubes, rectum, throat, eyes, joints, liver |
| Preferred Test | Swab or urine NAAT |
| Test Time to Results | Varies, 4–48 hours typical |
| Insurance | Broadly covers, recommended annually for women up to age 25 |
| Treatment | One-week course of antibiotics typical, alternative one-time dose |
| Partner Treatment? | Yes |
| Reportable? | Yes |
| Typically Found | Everywhere, all the time, increasingly throat and rectum |

I will end our discussion of chlamydia with this classic story of the flower child generation keeping up the reputation of enjoying free love and healthy sexual appetites. I'm all for enjoying the Golden Years, and I hope none of these anecdotes or lessons give the impression of shaming. There's nothing I like more than hearing about a healthy, active sex life in an older adult because, frankly, we should all be so lucky one day. Balancing the vigor with caution is the trick.

I was working as an ambulatory chief quality officer for a health system and my job was increasingly administrative. I was lucky enough to keep some clinical time at the STD clinic in the health department as well as keeping a small panel of primary care patients. When that clinic converted to an urgent care, I kept my little panel there and saw acute patients in between scheduled ones and partnered to support many of our advanced practitioners. Everyone knew of my love of STDs, so I would frequently get phone calls and texts in the midst of board meetings asking for advice on diagnosis and treatment and what to do in some of the messy, uncertain areas. I always took these calls. One call I received was from one of my favorite and more enthusiastic physician assistants.

"Dowler!" she exclaimed, "You will never believe what I just diagnosed!" (Insert dramatic pause for anticipatory tension to build.) "I just saw this super sweet 70-year-old lady who came in with vaginal discharge. It turns out she spent the weekend with her husband and another couple, and they were swingin'!"

"Define 'swinging,' please?" I asked.

"Dowler, they were all using the same sex toys and having sex with each other. They all have chlamydia! I am so glad I asked about her recent sexual history! Are you sexually active with men, women, or both? What body parts have been exposed to other people's body fluids? Do you ever trade sex for drugs or money?"

One of my firm teachings that I am adamant about is that taking a complete sexual history always pays off.

"If I hadn't asked, I probably would have figured she just had a yeast infection, but I took her full history, which led me to look for STDs, and I found the root of the problem!"

Too often in health care we are in such a hurry that we do not take the time to ask the extra questions that have the potential to unmask the diagnosis. At the same time, too often people will not disclose their full risks and exposures. In chapter 8 we will spend more time talking about how all of us could do this a little better.

### It's Tricky! Trichomonas

STDs are kind of like children: You aren't supposed to have a favorite. Despite this, I have a favorite STD. There, I said it. I'm sorry to all the other STDs, but the truth is out there. Trichomonas, at the end of the day, is simply my favorite. Why is that?, you are undoubtedly wondering.

> "It's Tricky"
> For some it begins as a trickle,
> Some men, when they pee, feel a tickle.
> The symptoms, they vary,
> So clinicians! be wary,
> Trichomonas is capricious and fickle.

Trichomonas is not actually a bacterium but a single-celled protozoan with whip-like flagella (sort of like tails). To understand the difference, you have to go back to sixth-grade biology. Essentially, the germ world is made up of bacteria, fungi, protozoans, and viruses. Chlamydia is a bacterium. Trichomonas is a protozoan. Yeast is a fungus. AIDS is a virus. All can cause genital infections but do so in different forms.

The accurate diagnosis requires a skilled clinician, and our historical "go to" test (a wet prep) is accurate only 50% of the time, making it a diagnostic challenge. A wet prep is when we take a swab of the vaginal discharge and place it in a test tube with a few drops of saline (water). We mix it together and then put a drop on a glass slide and place it on a microscope under magnification. This allows us to see what is happening in the vagina at a much higher level. The diagnosis of trichomonas was recently made easier due to advances in lab testing using the nucleic acid amplification tests (NAAT) that make gonorrhea and chlamydia so easy to diagnose, but many clinicians do not order this test, and many labs do not offer it locally, requiring it to be sent out to a distant lab. Send-out labs can be disruptive in the clinic—they require special swabs to be used, different orders and processes for the lab, and can take much longer since they are shipped somewhere else. Ergo, trichomonas often goes undiagnosed.

Until the recent NAAT advances, the diagnosis most often came in the form of a wet prep, which is useful only in women. Men just don't have an adequate supply of "juices" in a typical discharge to perform this test. Sadly, even with an experienced clinician, a diagnosis of trichomonas is missed half the time with a wet prep. Sometimes the trichomonads are dead so the classic "wiggling about" as the flagellum whip the organism in chaotic patterns around the slide is missed by the examiner, confused with other cells. When it is seen, though, it is infinitely gratifying and a little entertaining to watch. It is a little like watching a three-legged race. The movement is not graceful. For added dramatic flair, you can bring your patient to the microscope and show them what is causing their often-foul-smelling discolored discharge (always a crowd pleaser!). Even in a clinic that sees "trich" on a regular basis, when the clinician at the microscope calls out "trich!" everyone in the area can't help but stop what they are doing to glance into the microscope and watch the show.

In men, this organism is particularly challenging to diagnose because men will often not have the gross discharge of gonorrhea nor the urethral redness and subtle oozing of chlamydia. Often, they have no symptoms at all. If they have symptoms, they are usually subtle, describing "an itching feeling inside when I pee" or occasionally "a little burning in the middle of a pee" or even more rarely "a little crusting on my underwear." Trichomonas is very difficult to diagnose in men on exam. We cannot do a wet prep. The NAAT lab test is often not performed for a man as it is not part of the "normal screening" for many of clinicians. It is often missed until a woman gets the diagnosis.

Women who get infected with trichomonas, in my experience, are more likely to have symptoms. They will come in with a foul-smelling discharge and often describe it as greenish. It is possible they are having pain with sex. Many will have itching and have incorrectly treated it with an over-the-counter yeast medicine, which only creates more vaginal inflammation and discomfort. On exam they are frequently fairly inflamed, externally from the persistent discharge, and internally will have an angry, red cervix. The classic "strawberry" cervix, named for the appearance of the red, dotted fruit, is a giveaway. However, the frothy discharge is really what tells the story. An anaerobic organism, trichomonas releases a gas, and the discharge in the vaginal vault is often incredibly bubbly. Cheers! Women who have lower estrogen levels, such as women in or after menopause, are particularly vulnerable to trichomonas infection. Any vaginal discharge examination in a postmenopausal woman should definitely include ruling out "trich."

As I mentioned previously, of all the STDs with the possibility of infection without having had sex, while still incredibly unlikely, trichomonas is the one you would consider. It has been spread through sharing wet bath towels, loofahs, and even in pool water (but more on that later in the chapter).

Like chlamydia, the treatment for trichomonas is simple and straightforward—one dose of an antibiotic called metronidazole gets the job done (which will, incidentally, also clear giardiasis, should you drink a lot of creek water). Recent changes in guidelines recommends the dosing for women should be spread out over the course of a week for best results. Historically, this antibiotic was thought to have a wicked interaction with all forms of alcohol and causes violent vomiting and diarrhea. Based on old recommendations, if you are ever treated for trichomonas you should avoid alcohol for a full day prior to dosing and for a couple days afterward to avoid any complications, although recently released guidelines from the CDC did not find evidence to support that recommendation (table 4.2).

I had a young man in clinic once whom I diagnosed with trichomonas. It was a Thursday afternoon. I was explaining that he should abstain from alcohol until Sunday to be safe, and his eyes got wide. He asked if he could just wait to treat it until Monday.

"Why in the world would you delay treating your STD?" I asked. "Is it a problem to avoid alcohol for a couple days?"

(Red flag: Is he suffering from an addiction we need to explore?)

TABLE 4.2. Basics of trichomonas vaginalis

| Cause of Infection | *Trichomonas vaginalis, T. vaginalis* |
|---|---|
| Common Names | "Trich," TV |
| Type of Infection | Protozoan |
| Symptoms? | Variable, often in women |
| Duration of Infection | Weeks to years |
| What It Can Infect | Urethra, vagina, cervix |
| Preferred Test | Swab (females) or urine (males) NAAT preferred |
| Test Time to Results | Varies, 4–48 hours typical |
| Insurance | Broadly covers |
| Treatment | One-week course of antibiotics typical, alternative one-time dose |
| Partner Treatment? | Yes |
| Reportable? | No |
| Typically Found | Typically in heterosexuals |

"No, no, it's just that my girlfriend is coming to town this weekend, and I know we're going to be drinking, so I'd rather treat it after the weekend."

"Ah," I said. "So do you think you will be having sex?"

"For sure," he replied with youthful enthusiasm. "We don't get to see each other much, so we'll party all weekend!"

"Okay, so you don't want to treat the STD you got last week from a random hookup because you want to drink alcohol and have lots of sex with your girlfriend this weekend?"

"Right! I'll take the medicine on Monday," he affirmed, seemingly unaware of the problem with his reasoning.

I paused.

"So, you are going to infect your girlfriend with your STD this weekend in order to be able to drink with her?" I clarified, scrunching my face up with concern.

"Oh. Yeah. Right. Well, I guess we could use condoms . . ." he said.

"Condoms will protect her from infection but if the condom breaks or comes off, then all bets are off," I explained. "I wonder if you might go on and take the medicine today and skip drinking and sex this weekend. Maybe a nice hike instead?"

Interestingly, trichomonas is the only STD you will see predominantly in heterosexual relationships and rarely with men who have sex with men. It is implicated as a cofactor for HIV acquisition—in other words, if you have trichomonas and have sex with someone with HIV, you are more likely to get infected with HIV, possibly due to the inflammation the infection causes. Likewise, if you have HIV and another STD like trichomonas, you are more likely to transmit HIV due to increased viral shedding. Trichomonas also contributes to pre-term labor and low birth weights. It is the most rugged of STDs and is hardy—it can live on solid objects like sex toys and loofahs in the shower longer than most, certainly beyond 24 hours. You might be wondering: Can I get it from a toilet seat? Well, as I tell my teens, while theoretically it is possible, it would require the most unusual position-ing of the infected person and also the next person to use that toilet seat. It falls in the category of exceedingly unlikely. But there are cases where STDs can be transferred from person to person without sex-ual relations but via a shared inanimate object like a swimsuit.

One of my favorite tales to tell in my STD talks is that of the col-lege swim team that experienced an outbreak of trichomonas. Imag-ine the concern when a large number of the female swimmers all became infected. Were they all having sex with the same person? Were they all having sex with infected men? Were all the men in town carrying the same STD unknowingly? What in the world were these coeds up to?

The administration was horrified, the coaches mystified, the girls traumatized. Finally, after an investigation was concluded, the culprit was found: the swimsuit spinner (a device used to dry bathing suits off quickly). Yes, one infected young lady threw her swimsuit, freshly inoculated with vaginal discharge, into the spinner after practice. Sev-eral others followed, and the spinner spun the trichomonads in that warm, moist cylinder, contaminating all the swimsuits, which then transmitted the infection to their owners. Not only is this a tale of cau-tion when it comes to cleaning your swimsuit, but it is a fine story about the woes of rash assumptions.

## A Pox on Your House: Syphilis

One afternoon at the STD clinic, I saw a 69-year-old with a "rash" as the chief complaint, and my mind leapt to a few likely culprits. A pri-mary herpes outbreak was the most likely because of how much herpes we see in clinic. Second place in my mind was secondary syphi-lis, which presents with a rash, although most go to an urgent care or primary care assuming an allergic reaction. A molluscum contagio-sum outbreak was in distant third place—really unlikely but I like to have differential diagnoses in sets of three. (After 20+ years it becomes a sort of game to see how close I can come to guessing the diagnosis before seeing the patient and then after the labs come in.) This gentleman did not disappoint. Recently returned from a cruise, he explained how he and his partner enjoyed a very long monogamous marriage, with one exception. Every year they treated themselves to a gay cruise where they were free to explore sexual relations with anyone their hearts desired. His partner had received a call that he was a "contact to syphilis" from one of his cruise mates, so my patient felt he "better get checked to be safe." When someone is told they are a "contact to" it means one of their sexual partners has named them as a possible vector of infection, or as potentially newly infected. Interestingly, he had been to both his primary care provider and an urgent care about the funny rash he'd developed after the cruise, but no treatments had made a difference. He had tried antihistamines, topical and oral steroids, and antifungal medications without resolution. He admitted he had not shared his cruise activities mainly because "they didn't ask." When I asked him to turn up the palms of his hands, voilà! The classic palmar rash of secondary syphilis greeted me. Syphilis is one of only a handful (no pun intended) of infections—and the only sexually transmitted one—that will cause a rash on the palms of the hands or the soles of the feet.

> "Fridays in the STD Clinic"
> To tell you the truth, not being a prankster,
> But what else beats a big juicy chancre?
> With perhaps just a touch
> Of distal urethral pus
> Waiting at the end of an unguarded wanker.

Syphilis was one of my introductions to the world of "things that can go horribly wrong" in the young girl I saw in medical school, but at the time it was a relatively rare diagnosis. If you ran into it, it was invariably an old infection that had been brewing for many years. In fact, in 1999, the CDC announced a "Syphilis Elimination Plan" after seeing year-after-year declines in cases for over a decade. The end was, literally, in sight.

In the early 2000s, I made the diagnosis of secondary syphilis a few times, but the actual chancre of a syphilitic sore was something only to be imagined. Until, that is, the advent of hookup apps. Suddenly, in my urban mountain community we experienced an outbreak that lasted over two years related to anonymous partners on hookup apps. I was the envy of my STD colleagues—chancres abounded! No sooner had it settled down than it resurged again, but this time across the country.

Since 2014 we have seen steadily increasing rates of syphilis throughout the United States (fig. 4.1), most notably spread between men who have sex with men, but also accompanied by an increase in congenital syphilis (fig. 4.2). Congenital syphilis occurs when a pregnant mother infects the unborn baby with syphilis. In many states, screening for syphilis is compulsory for health care providers caring for pregnant women. Unfortunately, sometimes health care providers look at someone and determine they probably are not at risk. Even when they do all the right things, women might become infected between the time they have that screening test and delivery, by which point fetal devastation has already occurred.

One of my responsibilities in my role as chief medical officer for North Carolina Medicaid is to approve requests for home health services that exceed the insurance benefits' "normal" limits. I recently had to approve private duty nursing services for an infant. As I explored the child's medical history, I saw she had devastating neurologic limitations, intractable seizures, and had to be hooked up to a ventilator to stay alive, all from being infected with syphilis late in her mother's pregnancy. She would never live a normal life and would be lucky to survive past her fifth birthday.

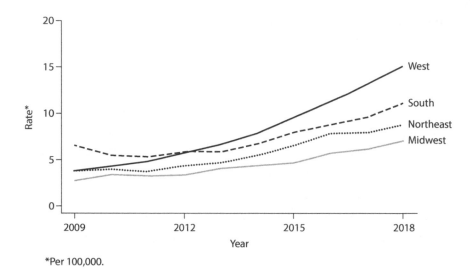

*Per 100,000.

FIGURE 4.1.

Rates of reported cases of syphilis by region of the United States from 2009 to 2018. *Source:* cdc.gov

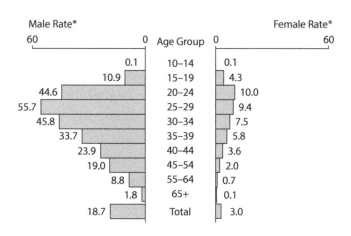

* Per 100,000

FIGURE 4.2.

Rates of reported cases of syphilis by age group and sex in the United States in 2018. *Source:* cdc.gov

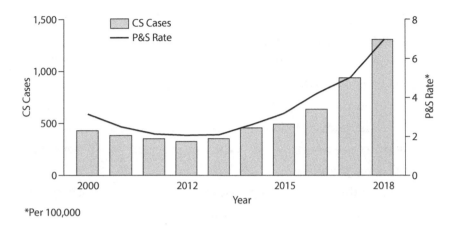

*Per 100,000

FIGURE 4.3.
Rise in congenital and primary and secondary syphilis cases
in the United States over time.
*Source:* cdc.gov

Why tell you about congenital syphilis if you are, in fact, past the reproductive age? How can I not? It is a public health crisis, and we should all be aware of those, whether they affect us directly or not. It's not "sexy," so it does not make the CNN 24-hour news cycle. You also might be part of a sexual network that could inadvertently share the infection and contribute to this tragic trend. What feels like an inconvenience to get a shot of penicillin to you is a life-or-death matter for someone else. Finally, if you are infected and don't notice the primary lesion, the progression of the disease is, in a word, awesome.

"Ah, Syphilis"
Our syphilis rate's gone through the roof
Believe me, y'all, I've seen the proof!
So keep your eyes peeled
Painless ulcers aren't feeled
Screen well for that moment of truth!

The first sign of syphilis is a painless sore, a "chancre" (pronounced *shank-er*). If it is in a place that is hard to see (the vagina, rectum), it is frequently never noticed. If noticed, many people will shrug it off, like one young man who thought the sore on his lip was just irritation from smoking too much since he was quite stressed out about a recent breakup. The primary lesion of syphilis is often missed by health care practitioners as well since many health care providers have never seen a case of primary syphilis.

If a syphilis infection progresses to secondary or tertiary syphilis, it can cause devastating consequences requiring hospitalization and repeated injections of penicillin. This progression can take months or years, so while someone does not know they are infected, they are spreading it widely while quietly damaging their own body.

"Rock On"
My inner STD princess is preening,
As my clinical obsession finds renewed
meaning.
The news, it's astounding!
Because syphilis is abounding,
USPSTF calls for more screening!

The resurgence of syphilis caused the CDC to release a "Call to Action" in 2017, leading to increases in screening recommendations and special advisories associated with increases in ocular and neurosyphilis. In these cases, patients present with vague eye symptoms that are often overlooked by a generation of health care providers who essentially forgot about syphilis.

There are three potential stages to a syphilis infection: primary, secondary, and tertiary. Each stage comes with increasing risk.

*Primary:* Indicated by a painless ulcer in mucosa, which resolves spontaneously in days to weeks.

*Secondary:* Symptoms include a vague, minimally symptomatic body rash, the "quintessential" palms of hand/soles of feet rash, and loss of hair in patches (alopecia).

*Tertiary:* This final stage can cause organ infection (such as in the brain or heart) and destruction of the brain (neurosyphilis), heart, and skin.

Testing for syphilis is very easy. The "screening" blood test, rapid plasma reagin (RPR), often stays positive once someone has had syphilis and is more likely to show false positives, so it is always advanced to a "confirmatory" test. The tables have turned in recent years, and what used to be done as the confirmatory test is sometimes now the first test and the other class of tests is run to confirm (called a reverse algorithm). Bottom line, the test results can be broken further down into four outcomes: a false positive (the person does not and has never had syphilis), prior syphilis (meaning the patient has had syphilis, but there is no evidence of a new infection), latent syphilis (meaning the patient has what is probably an old infection but not a new one), and active syphilis, which is self-explanatory. It can be very challenging to interpret the results of a syphilis test, so if your provider seems uncomfortable explaining the test results, forgive them. I cannot tell you how many times I have called the state STD services medical director to talk through a patient's presentation and subsequent lab results to develop a plan for treatment.

Treatment has been the same since penicillin was discovered. This is a remarkably easy infection to treat with a one-dose (for primary) injection of good old-fashioned penicillin. For patients allergic to penicillin, your health care provider will probably verify that you have a true allergy and not a sensitivity, because treatment becomes more complicated when penicillin is not on the menu.

### Gonorrhea: It's Nothing to Clap About

For Christmas a couple of years ago, my teenage son bought me a present that I still enjoy today: a T-shirt with "Gonorrhea, It's Nothing to

Clap About" in huge lettering on the front. He knows me so well! Gonorrhea has a lot in common with the other infections in this chapter. It can be asymptomatic (though less often than chlamydia, in my experience). It can infect the joints, eyes, skin, and all mucosa. It is incredibly contagious and requires a test of reinfection for high-risk patients. It can be diagnosed relatively rapidly, and if you are lucky enough to be in an STD clinic that does real-time gram stains, you can make the definitive diagnosis on the spot. However, there are a few things that make gonorrhea stand out: it has rapidly developed antibiotic resistance, so the treatment regimen changes often compared to other STDs, which can cause incomplete treatment from providers unfamiliar with handling sexually transmitted infections, and it can cause a truly impressive discharge from the penis.

"Hold the Applause, Please!"
Known by the famed moniker The Clap
Gonorrhea freely flows from the tap
Throat, anus, and joints
This infection appoints
With drug resistance a worsening trap.

There is a reason gonorrhea was historically called "the drip." Like a faucet left on just a tiny bit, the constant drip, drip, drip of gonorrhea is impressive to behold. Historically, in order to diagnose urethritis in a man, the clinician would do a gram stain and look under the microscope for the characteristic gram-negative diplococci. To do this, the clinician would insert a tiny swab into the urethra to gather a sample of discharge for investigation. This was not, for the record, particularly comfortable for the man and is a reason many men would avoid going to get tested. The good news is that now, the vast majority of the time, you can simply submit a urine specimen. What's different about gonorrhea is when someone is examined, there is no need to insert that little swab into the urethra because one can simply hold the microscope slide under the tip of the penis and a drop will plop down on the slide. (I know I don't actually need the gram stain confirmation when the discharge is abundant in this way, but I always do it to confirm and to see the lovely bright, pink-stained diplococci-filled cells peppering the slide.)

In women, gonorrhea is much sneakier and often asymptomatic or a surprise diagnosis on routine screening. For both men and women, gonorrhea is often present in the throat and rectum without symptoms, though it can cause symptomatic pharyngitis (infection of the throat) and proctitis (infection of the rectum). Much like the symptoms of strep throat, a patient with gonorrhea can complain about a sore throat, fever, and "white spots" (pus) on the tonsils. When the strep test is negative, an astute clinician will ask if you have had new oral sex partners (mouth to genital). But my guess is that it is not asked the majority of the time, so the diagnosis is often not made accurately. Despite guidelines to the contrary, many clinicians will give an antibiotic even with a negative strep test, perhaps unwittingly treating a gonorrhea pharyngitis. Rectal infection, while often silent with no symptoms, can cause proctitis, painful defecation (pooping), and rectal discharge.

Like chlamydia, gonorrhea can also infect the eyes. (Remember, this is not from eye sex!) One key difference is that when gonorrhea infects the eyes, it can rapidly progress and even cause blindness if not treated. Joints can also be impacted. Infection in a joint always requires immediate surgical debridement in the operating room. It has to be aggressively washed out to avoid permanent damage to the joint structures. Infection can also spread to the skin, and the patient will develop tender, red, pus-filled bumps.

The diagnosis of gonorrhea is relatively easy to make (table 4.3). It is immediate when you have gram stain microscopy in the office (usually only in STD clinics), but with the NAAT, test results are often available within 4 to 24 hours unless the test is shipped to a state lab or a distant reference lab. If someone has risk factors or if their exam meets certain criteria, the recommendation can be to treat the patient

TABLE 4.3. Basics of gonorrhea

| Cause of Infection | *Neisseria gonorrhea, N. gonorrhea* |
|---|---|
| Common Names | "The clap," "the drip" |
| Type of Infection | Bacterial |
| Symptoms? | Variable, many asymptomatic |
| Duration of Infection | Weeks to years |
| What It Can Infect | Urethra, vagina, cervix, fallopian tubes, rectum, throat, eyes, joints, skin, liver |
| Preferred Test | Swab or urine (male) NAAT, Gram stain from male urethral swab |
| Test Time to Results | Varies, 4–48 hours typical, Gram stain immediate |
| Insurance | Broadly covers, recommended annually for women up to age 25 |
| Treatment | Injection of antibiotic |
| Partner Treatment? | Yes |
| Reportable? | Yes |
| Typically Found | Increasingly found in throat, rectum |

"presumptively" while awaiting test results to prevent further spread. Treatment is theoretically quite simple, though it is complicated by the constantly moving target caused by the problem of antibiotic resistance (discussed in much more detail in chapter 3). This means sometimes clinicians are not aware of changes in the guidelines and will use an old treatment. This could cause a patient to have persistent infection, or the disease control team may reach out to them for appropriate treatment. Like chlamydia, often partners will not get treated or will time the treatments wrong, so reinfection is quite common. The combination of drug resistance and the chance for reinfection makes it very important to return for a repeat test of cure.

## Mgen: And Now for Something Completely Different

The newest bacterium in the hallowed halls of infected genitals is *Mycoplasma genitalium*—known colloquially as Mgen. Mgen was actually discovered several decades ago, but it is only recently coming into light as the cause of refractory (meaning persistent infection despite treatment) pelvic inflammatory disease and urethritis. It is also being credited with developing drug resistance even faster than gonorrhea. Unfortunately, it was not possible to diagnose this infection definitively until 2020, when the first FDA-approved NAAT test was released. This test is now slowly being accepted by insurers. (One of my first acts as CMO of NC Medicaid was to make sure we covered this test!) The United Kingdom is much further ahead with established diagnosis and treatment recommendations, while the CDC has still not issued formal screening, partner treatment, or diagnostic recommendations. Many clinicians have not yet put this bacterium on their radar of STDs because it is so newly implicated as a viable cause of significant genital infections, so do not be surprised if they seem skeptical when you ask about testing for this. While you should not ask for it as a screening test, if you are suffering from recurrent vaginal or urethral infections and your tests are all negative, make sure they have tested you for Mgen.

Like many of our other bacterial STDs, Mgen can be present for quite some time without any symptoms. On the other hand, it can also be present in someone with classic urethritis or cervicitis. It has been implicated as one of the major causes of pelvic inflammatory disease (PID), a condition present in younger women that can cause significant scarring of the reproductive pipes and lead to infertility long term. It is estimated that STDs, combined, contribute to infertility in 20,000 women in the United States each year. In the short term, like its STD cousins chlamydia and gonorrhea, Mgen can lead to hospitalization and time in the operating room for complicated pelvic infections as well. How many young women have we struggled to diagnose over the years who might have had Mgen?

In the late '90s, I was an intern on my hospital pediatrics rotation in the Bible Belt. This was during a time when virginity pledges were all the rage but the studies had not yet come out to illustrate the harms tied to them (as discussed in chapter 3). It was "RSV season." Respiratory syncytial virus is the cause of bronchiolitis (a lung infection) and was abundant in the community. The pediatric floor was overrun with infants suffering from this respiratory infection, which made them struggle to breathe or eat. One very memorable night while on call, I admitted 14 babies to the floor with bronchiolitis, setting a residency record.

Perhaps the "RSV fatigue" was the reason I so vividly remember the young girl that I admitted that night with abdominal pain—I was so excited to have something different on hand! At 14, she was a combination of passive and aggressive, with that classic on-edge energy the pubescent have when encountering authority. She was also in a lot of pain, which sharpened her defense mechanisms but made her vulnerable and lovable at the same time. In the late 1990s, the prevailing theory was to not treat abdominal pain with pain medications until you had a clear diagnosis, so that you did not throw off the exam, which in hindsight seems somewhat medieval. Her doting parents hovered, speaking with a thick Appalachian twang from outside of the city, and it was not long before I intuited that her father was a preacher.

The girl's CT scan came back, and I went to the bedside to discuss her probable diagnosis and why we needed to admit her to the hospital for surgery.

"Well, it is not appendicitis," I started, knowing the conversation was going to get very difficult very fast, because her infection was of the reproductive organs. She was young, from a very religious deep Appalachian family. The two did not go together well.

"Praise be!" her mother exclaimed, grabbing her daughter's hand.

Pale, the young girl was miserable, her eyes darting between her parents.

"It is not an ectopic pregnancy," I stated. "Her pregnancy test was negative."

"I reckon not," her father stated with narrowed, accusing eyes at the suggestion of such a thing.

"It appears she has a tubo-ovarian abscess and pelvic inflammatory disease," I began. "That means an infection has entered her uterus, her womb, and has moved up into her fallopian tubes and, on one side, the infection is surrounding her ovary."

"Lord help us. Bless your little heart," her mom murmured, patting her daughter on the hand. Meanwhile, her daughter looked increasingly anxious.

"How'd she get that? How do you fix it?" her father asked.

Awkward silence. Torn between full disclosure and protecting the patient, I waffled. "Well, sometimes this is from a sexually transmitted infection."

"She's never had sex!" Her father roared. "She's a child! So how else do you get it?"

"It's difficult to say, sir. We will need to do a pelvic exam and obtain some samples to send to the lab. Meanwhile, we will start IV antibiotics and plan to take her to the OR if the infection does not show signs of rapid improvement. The first order of business is to get her more comfortable with some pain medication."

In my mind, my cynical sleep-deprived eyes were rolling. Of course, she had had sex. And now she had an STD. And of course, she would never tell us her truth. With conservative parents like hers, how could she?

I remember her being on the pediatric floor for a prolonged hospitalization. She did require surgery and her recovery was slow. I have always wondered if she was ever able to bear children. That young lady never admitted to being sexually active. Her chlamydia and gonorrhea tests were both negative. Her intraoperative cultures were negative as well. Every day in rounds we puzzled over her case and never did solve it. In a quiet moment, I almost had a confession out of her, but her mother returned to the room just as I felt like we were going to have a breakthrough. With what I know now, I blame Mgen.

TABLE 4.4. Basics of *Mycoplasma genitalium*

| | |
|---|---|
| Cause of Infection | *Mycoplasma genitalium, M. genitalium* |
| Common Name | Mgen |
| Type of Infection | Bacterial |
| Symptoms? | Variable, many asymptomatic |
| Duration of Infection | Weeks to years |
| What it Can Infect | Urethra, vagina, cervix, emerging investigations |
| Preferred Test | Swab or urine (male) NAAT |
| Test Time to Results | Variable, 2–7 days though increasingly more available |
| Insurance | Broadly covers |
| Treatment | Two weeks of two antibiotics |
| Partner Treatment? | Yes, if positive |
| Reportable? | No |
| Typically Found | Increasingly found as cause of persistent urethritis/cervicitis/PID |

Since we have only very recently developed a test for Mgen and it was first mentioned vaguely in the STD Guidelines in 2015, this is truly a "hot off the press" STD (table 4.4). What we had previously done in the United States was treat the traditional infections, and if the symptoms resolved, even with negative tests, we were satisfied. We did not seek out partners and it was not reportable. (How can you report something you cannot actually test for?) If patients came back to the office with persistent symptoms, we would often do the same thing again (which, I believe, may be the definition of insanity—doing the same thing over and over and expecting a different outcome). Finally, if a patient met the diagnostic criteria for recurrent—or persistent—infection, we have in the past few years started treating presumptively for Mgen with a fairly aggressive antibiotic course.

With the advent of the recently FDA-approved NAAT test, there is hope for more direction for clinicians. More often than not, before this diagnosis is made, a patient has already had a trial of treatment with one or two other antibiotics. Currently, the most commonly recommended treatment involves a fairly aggressive course of a quinolone antibiotic, which has a significant side effect profile, including an increased risk for ruptured tendons. It is not recommended in teens or children and should be used with caution in older adults as well. After completing a course of a quinolone for a respiratory infection (not an STD), my own father ruptured his Achilles tendon when he was in his mid-60s. It resulted in a major surgery, a rehab stay, and a very long recovery. It is a great class of antibiotics, and when you need it, you need it—but it comes with risks.

The 2021 STI Guidelines has more guidance than in 2015, but there is not a wholesale recommendation for routine screening or asymptomatic partner treatment for Mgen. Between the difficulty in diagnosing and treating and the relative silence on guidelines, this is an infection many have never heard of—but mark my words, it won't be long before it grows much more well known. Think how savvy you will be to know about it (and avoid it) before others.

I will close this chapter on the treatable and curable sexually transmitted infections with this: It is a beautiful thing to tell a patient that you know what they have, and that you can treat it and cure it with the snap of your fingers. As we move into the chapters on the treatable but incurable and the potentially life-threatening or life-limiting infections, that sense of professional gratification is lost. These next two chapters bring the hard stuff.

## CHAPTER 5

# Treatable, Not Curable STDs

*All are on the scene, back in action,*
*Tear things up, put your parts in traction.*

JOHN WAS A NEAR-RETIREMENT ARTISAN who lived off the beaten path, several counties away from the local health department STD clinic he visited. His remote Appalachian community health department felt "a little too close to home," and he wanted anonymity in his care, so he would periodically hop into his road-worn pickup truck and make the drive over the mountain to visit me.

He had a long beard that straggled inches past his jawline and the teeth of someone who hadn't seen a dentist in many years. I wondered for a moment whether he might suffer from methamphetamine addiction, common in the Appalachian region, which has a devastating long-term effect on oral health. But John was all about clean living, except for his one vice. His fingers were stained dark from decades of heavy smoking, a companion he saw no future without. He was soft-spoken with a thick mountain accent, and I had to lean in and concentrate to make sure I understood what he was saying. Like many artisans, he was committed to his craft, and while he was not a wealthy man in dollars, he made up for it in the richness of his profession.

Over several years, John put a lot of mountain miles on that truck, and I spent an unusual amount of time up close and personal with his genitals. John had what I like to call "old school" genital warts—

heaping, rock garden, crusted, and cracked warts that are wide and thick and blanket the genitals like a well-worn quilt.

"John," I greeted him as he walked in one day. "Great to see you. How's work? Did you bring pictures? Warts come back again?" (For the record, you never *really* want to be on a chatty, first-name basis with an STD doctor.)

Despite my stern counsel, John would not quit smoking, which was the one thing that would have allowed us to stop meeting in the dark and damp basement of the health department. Smoking greatly increases the risk for recurrent and persistent genital warts. In countless creatively planned lectures during his wart treatments, when he was a truly captive audience, I would strategically accost him about his addiction.

"Here's the thing," I would say, firing up the apparatus that would freeze the thick warts until they got a frosty coating. "These warts will never clear up if you keep smoking. Never. You will grow old visiting me here." His reply would always be about how much he liked getting to see me, followed by him swiftly changing the topic. None of my usual tricks worked, not even suggesting he break up with his precious cigarettes once and for all with a "Dear John" letter (a clever joke if I say so myself!).

For months on end, I would see him every other Wednesday to freeze the warts and then paint on a toxic chemical (podophyllin) to hold the warts at bay and temporarily return his skin to a (relatively) normal appearance. He was uninsured and unable to pay the high price of a urologist for a more definitive laser treatment, so this was his best option. Sometimes months would go by before I would see him again, but he always came back.

John's addiction to nicotine was so great that he would endure repeated, painful, geographically inconvenient treatments of his genitals before he would even entertain the idea of quitting—the one thing that might have held his HPV infection at bay.

On one of his visits, I realized that I had become guilty of the one thing I chastised my colleagues about, and that was assuming he was not sexually active. Between his star-studded nether region and the amount of time it was blistered and oozing as it recovered from the wart treatments, it felt very unlikely he was sexually active, but I decided to refresh his sexual history. I asked my standard question: "In the last three months, have you been sexually active with men, women or both?" His answer truly surprised me, and I am hard to surprise!

"Just women, jeesh, Doc. You know I don't mess with men. Dang." Appalachian culture can lag at times on acceptance of diversity even among the relatively enlightened. He went on to reveal that he had been sexually active with a new female partner in the past month, and they were not using condoms. Remember, he was back in the clinic for his old-school genital warts that were so . . . big . . . they could have been named traveling companions.

"John, your girlfriend has sex with you without condoms?" I asked, horrified and perplexed.

He just shrugged and drawled, "I reckon she just doesn't look."

Little did he know, but John and his girlfriend were the inspiration for the catchphrase I use for my STD education, a phrase printed on keychain flashlights that I distribute to audiences when I give STD talks: "Lookie Before Nookie."™ My message to teens in particular is, "If you're comfortable enough with someone to have sex with them, you should be comfortable enough to scrutinize their genitalia!" For adults, this message also translates to taking the time to make sure your partner has a clean bill of sexual health. Do I think anyone is going to pull out a flashlight and do a formal genital exam before sex? No, I do not, though I am pretty sure I would if I ever hit the market again. My point is that before advancing to intimacy, you should at the very least be comfortable talking about prior infections, risks, and recent testing. You should definitely be aware if they are having a current outbreak of genital warts. Hopefully, this chapter about viral, treatable but incurable, uncomfortable, and undesirable STDs will drive this point home.

Viral STDs (caused by viruses) are my least favorite. Much like taxes, no one likes them and evading them is nearly impossible. They are highly contagious—of those who encounter them, few are spared. They are sneaky and elusive and stubborn. I really don't like viral STDs.

Let me tell you more about their wily ways. Many of the viral infections remain present even when there is no physical sign of infection. They can be difficult to definitively diagnose. They may or may not ever go away, and we have no ability to tell a patient whether they are still contagious. If you are lucky enough to vanquish these viral infections with your natural immune system prowess, you will literally never know. Are you beginning to understand my deep dislike for viral sexually transmitted infections?

According to the CDC, there were about 43 million HPV infections in 2018 in the United States alone, and nearly all sexually active people who do not get the HPV vaccine get infected with HPV at some point in their lives.

In May 2020, the World Health Organization released a study that showed that in 2016 almost half a billion (491.6 million to be exact) people in the world had genital herpes, and 3.7 billion (that's with a *B*) had oral herpes. Since herpes is a lifelong infection, the prevalence in their study showed increasing rates with age. Viral STDs are something you should care very much about.

Unlike bacterial STDs, which can be completely prevented with the use of condoms or other FDA-approved barrier methods, viral STDs can still spread through intimate contact on uncovered skin. This means the skin at the base of the penis into the groin and around the outside of the vagina and vulva, the areas that you can never completely cover with barrier methods, will always be exposed and at risk. This is a tough chapter because even people with the most cautious practices and the best of intentions can succumb to these infections.

We will focus on three viruses that plague the genitals: herpes, human papillomavirus (specifically the subtypes that cause genital warts—the ones that cause cancer will be covered in chapter 6), and molluscum contagiosum.

### Human Papillomavirus: Genital Warts

Tyrone was a middle-aged man who came into the STD clinic with an unusual complaint.

"Doc," he said, embarrassed and a little frightened, "I don't know what's happening but every time I pee . . ." he trailed off. He took a deep breath and looked away briefly and sighed. "Well, it sounds crazy but when I pee, instead of going in the bowl, it shoots out sideways and hits the wall! My wife's gonna kill me if I don't fix it, Doc."

"Interesting," I said, stalling because this was early in my STD career and I had no idea what was going on, though I will admit my first thought was mental illness. "Well, does anything look different about your penis? Any burning when you pee? Any changes you can see or feel?"

"No, it's all good."

"Hmm," I replied thoughtfully. (This is doctor speak for "Crap, what's going on?") "Any problems with sex function?"

"No."

"No new medicines?

"Nope."

"No change in products?" I asked almost desperately.

I was grasping. There's nothing that makes a new doctor sweat more than being face-to-face with a patient and having no immediate idea what's going on.

Suddenly, an idea came to me!

"Any trauma from sex?" I asked, thinking perhaps he had fractured his penis during an unusual sex position or some other trauma that had created scarring.

"Nope. It works fine. Normal. All good in that department. No problems."

"Well," I said, hopefully and perhaps weirdly enthusiastically, "let's just take a look and get some samples!"

Remember in chapter 4 when I said we used to have to do urethral swabs instead of urine samples on men? I saw Tyrone before urine tests were readily available, and this was one time when the swab came in handy. As I gently separated his urethral opening (the tip of the penis where the pee comes out) to insert the swab, peeking up to greet me was a genital wart hidden just inside his urethra.

Victory! I had solved the mystery of the sideways urination. His was a penis I will never forget. I can still see that pink shiny protrusion glistening in his lopsided urethra as if it was yesterday.

I pointed out the uninvited guest to Tyrone and explained, "You know when you use your garden hose and you put your finger over the end of the hose to create a spray? This wart is creating the same type of spray when you pee."

He was grateful to have an answer. I had never seen someone so relieved to discover an STD.

Tyrone's problem was fairly unusual. Often genital warts are more visible externally. But they can show up in a variety of locations. HPV is the single most common sexually transmitted infection in the United States today. Because it is not a reportable condition and because we do not have an easy in-office way to make a formal diagnosis in asymptomatic people, it is likely to be even more prevalent than we realize. HPV is so common that the CDC has made the bold statement that nearly all unvaccinated sexually active men and women will get the virus at some point in their lives.

HPV causes two things we care about: genital warts (this chapter) and cancer (chapter 6). Genital warts are unpleasant, but they will not kill you. Generally benign, these growths are caused by infection of the mucosa by certain subtypes of the human papillomavirus. They are caused by a different strain of HPV than plantar or palmar warts, which are also incredibly common but not sexually transmitted. Genital warts specifically infect genital mucosa, and while they will eventually go away, they are a cause of much embarrassment and significant discomfort if they are in a place that might experience trauma. One such place is the anorectal area, where warts can make wiping difficult and cause a desire to hold in bowel movements, which in turn can cause constipation, leading to tears of the tissue and impressive bleeding.

I have seen an array of strange and unusual things in the course of my career, but I recently hit a professional high. After 20 years of giving STD talks to teens and young adults, I experienced my first case of STD-induced syncope (fainting)! I was in my groove, waxing poetic about the many places in the human body that HPV can infect, when I noticed a slight commotion in the third row. The room had been darkened so I could project the infected genital pictures I've collected over the course of my career, and it was a little difficult to see what was happening back there. I noticed a faculty member walk up to the row and squat down, murmuring quietly, and then he and a boy walked out of the auditorium. It was not until after the presentation, when I asked the faculty what was going on, when I learned the boy had fainted. You might be wondering what exactly it was that did him in. What was the picture that caused this healthy male to slump out of his chair?

Anal warts.

It was a picture of a young man I had seen several years ago who had what can only be described as a small head of cauliflower growing from his rectum. This story is particularly poignant and memorable because he did not get it from anal sex with a man, which is the typical assumption. He got it from using his girlfriend's sex toy, which she had used first.

This is more common than you might imagine. One of my colleagues shared a story with me about two ladies in their mid-70s who came to the clinic together. One of them had a "breakout" of something, and her best friend was with her for moral support. As my colleague asked for a thorough sexual history (probably why she is one of my favorite colleagues—she's not afraid of a good sexual history), she learned that this started about a week after returning from a trip. The patient, her husband, her best friend, and her best friend's husband had taken a weekend trip down to Charleston. She realized she had left her vibrator at home, so she knocked on her friend's door and borrowed hers. Only a week later, she had her first outbreak of HPV, in her mid-70s. Interestingly, neither her friend nor her husband was aware of having HPV infection, but this is the exact kind of thing that makes me dislike viral STDs with such passion. They often last a lifetime and are completely asymptomatic.

Like many bacterial infections, HPV can also infect the mouth and tongue. The warts come in a variety of shapes and sizes, such as the "old school" warts, which are bigger and more prominent, and the newer warts, which are petite little mounds but can be shockingly numerous.

For reasons we do not yet fully understand, as was the case with our artisan, John, there is an interaction between the virus and smoking (or vaping) tobacco products that makes the virus much more difficult to treat and more likely to recur. Genital warts are oddly persistent, whether they are in the mouth, the butt, or the penis or vagina. Even after someone has genital warts treated and the skin looks clear, they can still shed the virus from the skin, infect others, and have recurring infections. Smoking makes this pattern of recurrence much more likely to happen, with the hypothesis that smoking weakens the immune system and creates more vulnerability to infection.

Pregnant women who already have genital warts, or who get them during pregnancy, will often see a fairly significant blossoming of the infection during their pregnancy—enough so that sometimes we will elect for a C-section to avoid the trauma of tearing the tissues (which are difficult to sew back together). HPV infection acquired through traumatic sex also can result in significant outbreaks. The worst case of genital warts I have ever seen was in a nonpregnant, non-immune-suppressed eighth-grade girl who had been sexually assaulted by several of her "friends." They were drinking alcohol after a school event, and she drank so much she did not remember much of the experience. She would not consent for me to connect her to resources like the police, a therapist, or a support group, and she was of an age to make her own health care decisions based on her sexual activity. While she was very much a minor, the age of consent for making health care decisions in North Carolina is 13. Her shame was so great that she refused to name the perpetrators or even tell her parents. This was in the early 2000s, well before the #MeToo movement, and I could not change her mind, despite repeated efforts. She was one of the most impressive young women I have ever met in a clinical setting. She came back to the clinic, week after week, stoic and determined, so we could freeze and chemically burn the dozens of genital warts until they finally resolved. The good news today is that the treatment for genital warts has improved with time.

While we cannot cure genital warts, modern medicine can make them go away with less pain and inconvenience than ever before. There is a highly effective prescription cream that can be applied to the warts from the comfort of home by patients over the course of several weeks. For many years, this type of cream was so expensive that many of the patients I cared for chose not to go that route. But today there is a generic version available, and it is the treatment of choice for most patients. After 6 to 12 weeks of home treatment, the warts usually resolve (unless you are a smoker, and then all bets are off). If the warts don't resolve, it's important to follow up with your health care provider because you may need to have the skin biopsied to rule out a type of skin cancer. Anyone with an STD should have routine screening tests performed for other infections. It is particularly important to make sure you have had a syphilis test because secondary syphilis, which we learned about in chapter 4, can cause "condyloma latta," which can be visually confused with genital warts.

> "Waxing and Waning"
> Genital warts are more waning, less waxing
> Could the scourge of HPV be relaxing?
> Well, pull out that shot,
> Immunize the lot!
> That vaccine makes our clinics less taxing!

What is even better than treatment? Prevention! While condoms and other barrier methods decrease your chance of getting HPV infection, they are not a guarantee. In 2006, the HPV vaccine was introduced, and STD health care providers were ecstatic. The guidelines stated that all 12- to 13-year-old girls were to get the series of vaccines (developed primarily to prevent cervical cancer, which I share more about in chapter 6). The idea at the time was that herd immunity would protect the men, since women were more likely to harbor the infection for long periods of time. In other words, if the girls could not get it, the boys would not get it. Finally, STD health care providers around the world proclaimed, the end of these bottoms covered in warts! No more teens collapsing in a puddle of tears because they hadn't realized that being with four partners in three months meant a very high chance of getting or sharing this virus. My days of getting up close and personal with infected bottoms in order to paint an acid ever-so-carefully onto the rough surface of warts but not the healthy mucosa surrounding them were going to end! Victory party!

Fast forward to what actually happened.

The religious right did not support a vaccine for teens related to sex because they claimed it would encourage promiscuity. This was also the time when falsely published research outcomes were creating a generation of anxious parents who were certain that vaccines would cause autism in their children. The media and anti-vaxxers got on the scene with horrific tales of teens "dying" from the vaccine (which, to be clear, was completely untrue). Parents and health care providers alike became hesitant. Shouldn't they just wait until the 12- and 13-year-olds were a little older before giving them the vaccine?

Pause for science: The vaccine was being given at that age because there were concerns it might not be as effective after "Little Sally" had sex the first time, so it was better to fully vaccinate her before that window closed. With one in three women contracting an HPV infection with their sexual debut at that time, waiting created the risk of missing an opportunity for prevention. And let's be honest, what doctor hasn't delivered the baby of a 13-year-old? Kids choose to have sex when they want to have sex; in addition to this, they are also victims of assault more often than we would like to imagine.

Vaccine uptake was low initially. Not just low: it was subterranean. But over time, we have been able to dispel the myths around the risk of death or autism. The "deaths" were more about teenagers passing out after the vaccine because it hurt, and tragically, when someone passes out, they might hit their head and even die. We learned that by having the teens lie down for 10 minutes after the vaccine, that time of vasovagal syncope (the medical terminology for this fainting) will pass and they will be fine. The recommendations and dosing have also changed several times in the past 15 years as research has taught us more. To date, the HPV vaccine appears to provide lasting, long-term immunity, and distribution has since been expanded to include boys as well as girls. You can believe my teen boys got their vaccine the minute the guidelines said they could. The guidance has even been extended to say that the vaccine can still be given after your sexual debut. Insurance companies began measuring the quality of a health care provider's care years ago based on their following of evidence-based guidelines—and for many payers, this includes the HPV vaccine.

The strength of evidence that it can prevent cancers is just that overwhelming. Even many adults are now able to receive the vaccine.

Slowly but surely, vaccine uptake has increased (fig. 5.1), and the flow of patients whom I get to know really well because of week after week of genital freezing has slowed to a trickle. However, despite these efforts, at present only 49% of adolescents have received the complete vaccine series.

That means that over half of teens and young adults are partially, or completely, vulnerable to infection that could lead to cancer. You are probably wondering if you should get the vaccine. If you are as old as me, I'm afraid not. The guidelines clearly state that the vaccine is indicated up to age 45, as it is not FDA approved for older populations at this time. Thus far, drug companies have not paid for studies in older adults. If you would like to read more on the current guidelines, the American Cancer Society published a helpful resource, "Human

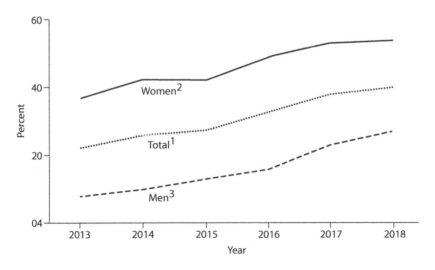

FIGURE 5.1.
Percentage of adults aged 18 to 26 who ever received one or more doses of human papillomavirus vaccine, by year and sex in the United States from 2013 to 2018.
*Sources:* NCHS, National Health Interview Survey, 2013–2018;
https://www.cdc.gov/nchs/images/databriefs/351-400/db354_fig1.png

Papillomavirus Vaccination 2020 Guideline Update," *CA: A Cancer Journal for Clinicians* 70, no. 4 (2020): 274–80, https://doi.org/10.3322 /caac.21616.

Even though you can't get the vaccine yourself, you still can use barrier methods such as male and female condoms and dental dams to help protect yourself from HPV (table 5.1). You can also reach out to your kids, grandkids, and great grandkids and ask them if they have had the HPV vaccine. If they have not, encourage them to. Not only are you saving them from the embarrassment of unsightly warts on their wee parts, but you might be protecting them from cancer down the road.

## Herpes Simplex Virus

I spent time doing shifts in an urgent care facility when my children were very young. My husband traveled internationally for work, and my full-time health department job was wonderful, but every time

TABLE 5.1. Basics of human papillomavirus

| | |
|---|---|
| Cause of Infection | Human papillomavirus, >100 benign subtypes |
| Common Name | HPV |
| Type of Infection | Virus |
| Symptoms? | Variable, asymptomatic, warts, invasive cancer |
| Duration of Infection | Lifetime |
| What It Can Infect | Urethra, vagina, cervix, rectum, anus, mouth, tongue, lips, throat |
| Preferred Test | HPV testing on cancer screening/diagnosis only |
| Test Time to Results | N/A |
| Insurance | Broadly covers cervical cancer screening |
| Treatment | Warts: variable, topical home treatment or in-office treatment |
| Partner Treatment? | No |
| Reportable? | No |
| Typically Found | Everywhere, all the time |

Jared would leave the country one of the boys, then 2 and 4, would somehow get sick or injured. This would result in canceling a full day (or even days) of patients, which was inconvenient for everyone. At the time, the county would not allow part-time work.

One of my best friends and colleagues who worked with me was undergoing breast cancer treatment and was committed to staying, and we proposed a job share. No dice. Sadly, both of us left the health department for part-time employment. The urgent care where I signed up for shift work was nonprofit with Catholic-based ownership and had a generous charity care program, so the move from public health to treating underserved populations was not as painful as it might have been. I remained at the STD clinic a couple days a week while working two or three 12-hour shifts a week at an urgent care site where STDs were almost as common as sinus infections. There is something about the anonymity and spontaneity that the walk-in, after-hours environment offers that brings patients from all walks of life to an urgent care instead of their primary care doctor or advanced practitioner for many STD complaints.

The chief complaint on the patient's chart that I picked up was "pain with urination." Got it. Quick, easy, UTI. I figured I'd be able to take care of her and then grab lunch in the break room before the evening crowd pulled up. Without fail, mid-to-late-afternoon in this urgent care would be slow, and then it seemed as if a bus had pulled up and dropped off dozens of people every evening to keep us hopping until we locked our doors for the night.

I went into the room and was greeted by an elegantly attired older woman who said she was in town for horseback riding with friends. She sat uncomfortably, and I was not sure if it was because of our unglamourous surroundings (she was distinctly out of place) or from pain.

"I'm sorry to say that after our first ride, I started having this terrible pain with urinating," she explained formally. "It has simply become unbearable. I hold it as long as I can to avoid the pain." She explained that she felt like she might be running a fever as well. The nurse had obtained a urine sample before I went into the room, and it was already on the chart: high white blood cells (a sign of infection) and blood, possibility from infection, trauma, or menstrual bleeding.

It would have been easy to say "UTI," prescribe an antibiotic, and send her off to her travel companions, but something in the way she was sitting made me ask another question.

"Have you noticed any other symptoms in your vaginal or vulvar area?"

She shifted uncomfortably on the hard plastic chair. "Well, yes, actually. I have been having some swelling down there for a couple of days. It's made it very uncomfortable to ride."

She agreed to an exam, and I had one of those moments when my mouth works faster than my brain: as I looked at her perineum, I exclaimed, "Oh my gosh! You poor thing!"

Her vulva was a minefield of ulcers, her labia swollen almost completely together. How she was able to walk, much less ride a horse, was beyond me. She was having her first herpes outbreak.

What's the difference between love and herpes?
Herpes lasts forever!

Herpes: the nemesis of health care providers everywhere. Herpes is a pain in every way—most notably for the people with ulcers on their sensitive parts, but it is also a terrible diagnosis to share with a patient. There is no good way to tell someone that they may have recurring, painful genital lesions for the rest of their lives, will be infectious to everyone they have sex with, and are at increased risk for getting other sexually transmitted infections, like HIV. On top of all those reasons to dislike herpes, it can also present real diagnostic and prognostic challenges to even the most experienced clinician.

Earlier, I shared that 1 in 5 people have genital herpes. Like HPV, it is an infection that is not reportable, and, as I shared previously, it is challenging to diagnose. Those combined factors suggest that in reality, more than 1 in 5 people are infected. In fact, a study published in 2016 by the World Health Organization reinforced the previously established data that as many as 9 out of 10 adults infected with genital herpes either do not know it, have such mild symptoms they have never sought a diagnosis, or are oblivious to their diagnosis. When you look at the global incidence of herpes, the United States comes in second place, only behind Africa, for the prevalence of this infection.

Herpes is an infection that does not discriminate based on age, and if anything, I have seen more older adults develop it in recent years than ever before. While most new infections are in adolescents, prevalence increases with age, so the majority of people living with herpes are older adults. Like HPV, herpes has more than one subtype. You will remember that HPV has well over 100 subtypes but only two strains that concern us: the ones that cause genital warts and the ones that cause cancer. Herpes also has two predominant subtypes we are concerned about: type 1, "oral" herpes and type 2, "genital" herpes. Historically, the majority of people are infected with type 1 sometime in their formative years—as many as 80% of children develop "stomatitis" (an inflammation or sore inside the mouth, usually on the tongue, cheeks, gums, or the interior of the lips). The infection will spread through a preschool or kindergarten class like wildfire.

I remember my son, Jacob's, bout of stomatitis the week before starting kindergarten. His mouth was peppered with shallow, inflamed ulcers so painful he avoided swallowing his own saliva. We were at the beach when he developed a fever and sores, days after preschool "graduation." He would not eat or drink, and I became increasingly concerned, he would soon need IV fluids to treat his dehydration. All four of us (Eli was 3 at the time and had not yet succumbed) squeezed into the car and drove for hours trying to find an urgent care (we were in an isolated coastal town, and this was well before the advent of the smartphone or Google Maps). We finally gathered enough local intel to realize that our only option was to drive to Wilmington to an emergency room, but miraculously, the long drive had lulled Jacob into a drooling stupor. Instead of going to the emergency room, we went to a store and bought every desirable soft or liquid item we could find and plied him with these treats until the crisis passed.

I tell you this story to illustrate the point that type 1 herpes—the infection of the mouth—is ubiquitous in school settings. What is different today, interestingly, is that fewer young people are exposed to type 1 herpes infection, so they don't have immunity to it. When they are exposed by someone with type 1 herpes, they can then get the infection in their genital areas. Because of this, we are beginning to see a crossover of oral and genital infections in sexually active adults. Why is that?

The sequelae (the enduring effects) of that type 1 infection that is so common in childhood are the subsequent "fever blisters" that show up around the edge of the lip and wreak havoc on prom pictures. You will remember that a herpes infection is lifelong; once infected, you will remain infected and continue to shed the virus. Many people have recurrent outbreaks over the course of their lifetime. Fever blisters can be triggered by a wide variety of insults: weather exposure (a day of skiing), physical trauma (trimming a mustache), physical stress (fever), hormones (menses), and emotional stress (final exams). Recurrences vary from person to person. Some people will never have an outbreak, and some have so many they take medicine daily to prevent it. Before an outbreak, the majority of people will experience a "prodrome"—a subtle sign that a blister is coming. For most it is a tingling, itching, or burning sensation of the skin in the area where the outbreak will occur. Luckily, there is a class of antiviral medicines that is very effective, and most people learn the clues early on and can start the medicine at the very first sign, thus preventing a full breakout.

Here is a great teaching moment: Anyone with obvious cold sore outbreaks should avoid giving oral sex during that time of high virus shedding. But you may wonder, what if you only have outbreaks every now and then? Are you still shedding virus all the time and potentially infectious? Unfortunately, yes. Barrier methods are important to decrease the risk of transmission to others.

Type 2 herpes has historically been considered genital herpes, as in the case of the horseback rider earlier in the chapter. Like type 1, the first outbreak is significantly worse than subsequent outbreaks. In fact, everything about type 2 is worse than type 1. Many people will develop a flu-like illness up to a week after their infection: fevers, body aches, headache, and fatigue. Most will develop tender, swollen lymph nodes that feel like grape-sized swellings in the groin.

The typical "course" of a genital herpes infection and subsequent outbreaks is fairly predictable. For most people, the prodrome will occur after the initial infection—that itching, burning, or tingling of the skin in the area where a blister will next appear. The blister is the first visible sign, and there can be as few as one very subtle blister or dozens and dozens of blisters. These are fluid-filled bumps that people notoriously try to "pop," assuming them to be ingrown hair, which of course then creates an oozing of fluid filled with a gazillion viruses standing ready to infect. After the blister(s), the skin necroses (dies) and an ulcer develops in place of the blister. These are typically very red with a shallow base and are quite painful, with tiny nerve endings tightly packed into the genital tissue that is exposed to the outside world. Eventually the ulcer will form a scab or crust, and then the outbreak will resolve. This can happen in as few as a handful of days, or it can take weeks. And remember, many do not have outbreaks and so do not know they are infected.

Some people will be infected in their urinary tract and develop urinary tract symptoms, referred to as "hematuria-dysuria syndrome." Urinalysis will show white blood cells and microscopic blood (blood cells that can be seen with high magnification but not by the naked eye), and this can be mistakenly diagnosed as a UTI. However, when the urine is sent for a culture to identify the bacteria causing the infection, the culture does not grow out bacteria. By the time the culture is resulted back as negative, the patient will have finished an unnecessary course of antibiotics, and the herpes will have resolved. This can happen recurrently, especially in patients who see a variety of different health care providers who never put together the urinary symptoms and negative cultures.

In severe cases, the patient can develop encephalitis (infection and inflammation of the brain) and require hospitalization; a study published in the *Journal of Critical Care* revealed that as many as 70% of patients will die from a herpes encephalitis that is not accurately diagnosed and treated. However, this is unlikely to happen with our current level of rapid diagnostic testing, and the death rate today is only 5%.

Typically, in the first year following a genital herpes infection, the patient will experience the most severe and frequent outbreaks. Over time, the frequency and intensity diminish for most. Unfortunately, with age, the immune system can weaken; major insults to the body, like a severe pneumonia, can result in an outbreak of an infection that has lain dormant for decades.

One of the challenges with a herpes diagnosis is that much like warts, outbreaks come in all shapes and sizes. I can't tell you how many people have come into the clinic for me to look at their "razor burn" or "maybe I got my penis stuck in a zipper" or "I think I scratched myself masturbating" to diagnose a primary herpes outbreak. To the eye that has seen more herpes outbreaks than sunsets, it's an obvious diagnosis, but to the untrained eye it just looks like a break in the skin. Add to this that quite often the blister or ulcer is in an area that is difficult for an arthritic or inflexible person to see, and so will resolve without treatment, and it is easy to understand why many people are never diagnosed. Other people experience horrific outbreaks with countless ulcers on their most sensitive areas. Every person's experience is different, so you shouldn't assume that your outbreak will just go away without having it looked at by a professional.

Women are prone to having outbreaks in the perirectal area (true also of HPV) even if they have never had anal sex. This is because of gravity and body fluid drainage that naturally flows down. When a woman is supine (lying on her back) and fluids ooze, gravity takes them to the perirectal area, where they can infect the more southern regions of the perineum (the area between the vagina and the anus). The same can be true of those who receive oral–anal sex: they can develop type 1 perirectal herpes infection even without experiencing penetrative anal sex.

In the past, the only way we could diagnose herpes definitively was with a culture that could take months to yield a result and required very specific storage and handling. In clinic, we would "unroof" a blister (gently lift the top layer of skin to expose the fluid) and use a swab to pick up ulcer juice and send it off to grow in special media. If transport went well and we were able to get a nice sample, a result would come in a few months later. For that test to work, the person needed to come into the office when they had a juicy blister that had not yet turned into an ulcer. The problem was that people often delay health care—due to denial, lack of insurance, busy lives, or because their special health care provider is not available—until the ulcers are at their peak and the discomfort becomes unbearable. That often meant no more juicy lesions to culture and a diagnosis that was a presumption. For some, that was enough for the power of denial to convince them it was not really herpes. The slowness of the old culture method translated to agonizing months for someone to wait for a diagnosis and a high risk of a "false negative" test.

Today, we have much better options. We can still do a culture, but in 2000 PCR technology, which is much more advanced, was developed. This is now commercially available in routine labs, so we can also take a sample directly from a lesion that yields results much more quickly than culture. While there has been a very basic blood test for a long time, it did not differentiate between type 1 and type 2. Since so many people have type 1 from childhood and have no memory of it and no recurring cold sores, that meant positive tests were very hard to actually interpret and you could not tell someone if they had both types (1 and 2), or if they were only positive from an old childhood infection. It really only created increased anxiety for patients.

The newer herpes blood test (an immunoglobulin type-specific test) can tell the clinician whether the patient has been infected with type 1 and/or type 2. It has been a fantastic development, since so many people are asymptomatic or minimally symptomatic with infection. However, it does have limitations—for instance, it will only be positive after time has passed since the infection. This can vary depending on the severity of infection and a person's immune response, but I recommend people wait at least six weeks after exposure. If someone rushes to the health care provider for a test right after a high-risk exposure or early symptoms of infection, the test will say "negative" even when there is a new infection brewing. People read the news stories about herpes being common and they want to know if they have it, so they ask for the blood test, but it is intended for definitive diagnosis, not screening. Every lab test has its limitations and performs best when used in a population with a higher risk of infection. The same is true for this blood test, and the CDC does not recommend using it for routine screening for herpes infection.

One reason for this is how difficult it can be to interpret the results for patients. We know that most people had type 1 herpes in childhood, so if the test comes back positive for 1, what do you do about it? Is it a type 1 oral infection or a type 1 genital infection? We have also seen increases in type 1 outbreaks in the genital area over the past two decades, so is a positive type 1 just an old oral infection or a new genital infection?

What if you are positive for type 2 but have never had a genital outbreak? Now what? Are you contagious to everyone forever? Based on our knowledge today, the answer is yes. Using the blood test for screening for herpes in the absence of symptoms or known exposure ends up with more questions than answers, and it can be frustrating for all parties involved.

So, who should get the herpes test? The CDC has clarified its recommendations in the 2021 STI screening guidelines. I will share how I recommend clinicians use the herpes immunoglobulin type-specific blood test for screening asymptomatic patients who desperately want the test, based on my clinical experience:

- *High Risk:* Herpes, like trichomonas, serves as a co-factor for HIV acquisition. Knowing you have herpes if you are a high-risk individual can provide important information on your risk of getting HIV. Therefore, men who have sex with men and are not in long-term monogamous relationships may benefit from testing. The same is true for IV drug users, sex workers, and women who have sex with men who have sex with men. Frequent hook-up app users fall into this category as well. However, the question of how often a test should be done remains, because each new partner opens the door to a new infection. Therefore, this assessment must be made based on each individual patient's habits.
- *New Infection:* When Partner 1 in a couple is diagnosed for the first time with herpes and Partner 2 is now terrified (that they gave it to Partner 1 or will get it from Partner 1), it can be helpful

to find out if Partner 2 came into the relationship with herpes. Whenever someone has an STD, they invariably become desperate to know who "gave it to them." In this situation it is not about blame. Rather, it is about whether Partner 2 is now at risk. If both partners are positive for both 1 and 2, then using barrier methods 100% of the time is not necessary. The cat's out of the bag, so to speak.

• *Known Infection:* When a new relationship is ready for the next step and Partner 1 knows they have had herpes in the past, it can be helpful for Partner 2 to have testing. As in the above scenario, if they are infected and just didn't know it, the risk of becoming infected becomes moot. If Partner 2 is negative, there is good evidence that transmission can be prevented if Partner 1 takes the prescribed antiviral medicine every day and they use condoms 100% of the time. It is important for the couple to have the chance to make this choice together.

> "Making the Diagnosis"
> They regret going past the full flirting
> Now their wee bits sure are hurting.
> Mind full-on churning
> Bottom, blistered, burning
> The news devastates, disconcerting.

Perhaps the most complicated part of herpes today, aside from the diagnostic challenges and people not being aware they are infected, is sorting out type 1 from type 2. We are increasingly seeing type 1 genital infections and less often type 2 oral infections, and the "historical" anatomical divide between the two has been almost completely eliminated. Overall, type 2 is much more likely to be genital, and generally most genital infections are type 2. Here are some of the most common questions I get about type 1 and 2 herpes. The permutations are endless! (Well, not really endless, per se.)

**Q:** What if someone with type 1 herpes on their mouth has oral sex with someone who does not have herpes?

**A:** The person who is receiving the oral sex may get type 1 herpes on their genitals. This happens all the time.

**Q:** What if someone gives oral sex to someone with type 2 herpes?

**A:** They may get type 2 herpes on their mouth.

**Q:** What if someone receives anal sex from someone with a history of type 2 herpes?

**A:** They may get type 2 perirectal herpes.

**Q:** What if someone uses a sex toy from someone with a history of type 1 genital herpes?

**A:** They may get type 1 genital herpes.

Herpes is a challenge for patients and clinicians alike (table 5.2). It can be devastating when you make that diagnosis. It has been the

TABLE 5.2. Basics of herpes

| | |
|---|---|
| Cause of Infection | Herpes simplex virus type 1 and 2 |
| Common Names | HSV, herpes |
| Type of Infection | Virus |
| Symptoms? | Variable, many asymptomatic |
| Duration of Infection | Lifetime |
| What It Can Infect | Urethra, vagina, cervix, penis, anus, rectum, mouth, lips, throat, eyes, liver, brain |
| Preferred Test | PCR or culture from lesion, NAAT blood (Glycoprotein G 1/2) |
| Test Time to Results | Days to months |
| Insurance | Broadly covers |
| Treatment | Symptoms managed with oral antiviral medication |
| Partner Treatment? | No |
| Reportable? | No |
| Typically Found | Everywhere, all the time |

cause of more tears than any other STD I have diagnosed. The potential of a lifelong infection that may be shared with every partner the patient encounters is the real grief of a herpes diagnosis. Like with HPV, condoms help, but they cannot prevent transmission, so the diagnosis feels life-altering to many. However, with our improvement in the use of oral antiviral medications, the symptoms can be kept at bay, so the physical discomfort of herpes is no longer the biggest hurdle to overcome, and the virus can be meaningfully suppressed. The data are also very clear—many adults walking around are already infected with genital herpes and have no idea.

## Molluscum Contagiosum

Amanda came into my clinic complaining of "bumps" on her mons pubis (the fatty mound in front of the pubic bones). She was a sophomore in college and stated that she had absolutely no risk factors for STDs. She was not currently and had never been sexually active. She did not drink or smoke or do drugs. She worked hard in school and endured typical college stress but had no other concerns.

She had developed two bumps that she thought were ingrown hairs. She did shave all of her pubic hair regularly, and the bumps were on the skin up high, well above her clitoris. She tried popping them, but instead of going away they began spreading. The more she popped the more they spread. She had looked on the Internet and was worried she had genital warts but could not understand how she had gotten them.

A couple decades in the STD clinic will make anyone a cynic, and I suspected her self-diagnosis was right before I examined her.

"Define 'not sexually active,'" I said with a raised eyebrow. How many times had I asked someone if they were sexually active, and they had said no but then went on to say they'd last had sex a few days ago? "Active" is in the eyes of the beholder.

"No sex. Ever." She was emphatic. She made eye contact.

Okay, I thought, maybe her claim was legit, but I still needed to specifically ask to be sure. "Oral sex? Anal sex? Sex toys?" I asked, just to be certain. She denied all of it.

I left the room while she changed and pondered how I could explain HPV in someone who had never had sex. She also denied sharing juicy sex toys, but that was a remote possibility. It was going to be a hard sell.

I returned to the room and examined her. She had dozens of tiny bumps on her mons pubis, which had been shaved clear of hair. Some were scabbed over. Others had a red base and were fluid-filled blisters. Herpes, I wondered? No, they clearly were not painful when I poked at them. I asked my nurse for a magnifying glass and looked closer, and I was delighted to find a dimple in the middle of several lesions.

"Molluscum contagiosum!" I declared enthusiastically.

Relieved it was not HPV or herpes, I proceeded to explain the diagnosis of molluscum contagiosum to her. After an extensive medical history and sleuthing expedition, we came upon the most likely culprit—a tanning bed. She had recently started tanning. She always lay prone and unclothed, and she had not been wiping down the beds before climbing in. Add to that her regular shaving of the pubic region, and the microscopic cuts in the skin that result, and you have the perfect entry for an ill-timed, unanticipated exchange of body fluids.

I will end chapter 5 with the good news that there *is* a viral STD that is not a big deal! For those of you familiar with molluscum, you are probably wondering how this fairly benign and annoying virus that plagues children can be an STD. Well known to parents of young children, molluscum is a ubiquitous virus in the halls of preschools and elementary schools. Both of my children battled it during childhood. It is not thought of as a "classic" STD because the majority of infections are not sexually transmitted, but when it appears in the genitals or oral mucosa of an adult, it is almost always transmitted sexually.

TABLE 5.3. Basics of molluscum contagiosum

| Cause of Infection | *Molluscum contagiosum, M. contagiosum* |
|---|---|
| Common Name | Molluscum |
| Type of Infection | Virus |
| Symptoms? | Typical skin lesions |
| Duration of Infection | Weeks to months |
| What It Can Infect | Labia, penis, skin |
| Preferred Test | Rarely indicated |
| Test Time to Results | N/A |
| Insurance | Broadly covers treatment |
| Treatment | Topical home treatment, in-office treatment |
| Partner Treatment? | No |
| Reportable? | No |
| Typically Found | School-aged children, occasionally as STI |

The classic presentation is bumps that someone always tries popping, thinking they are zits or ingrown hair. People do this even where hair doesn't typically grow. They can't help themselves! When they pop the lesions, it makes them spread further. Any sort of irritation, like shaving, will also contribute to the spread. Sometimes people will complain of a mild itch, but for many there are no symptoms at all.

Like HPV, molluscum will eventually go away on its own after weeks or months. Unlike HPV, it does not have the potential to lead to complications like cancer, and there is no evidence that this virus will likely come back—so once it is resolved, you are no longer infectious. The exception to this is someone with severe immune suppression, such as those with AIDS or who have had a solid organ transplant. In these patients the infection can be devastating, but for the average person, it falls into the "brief and time-limited nuisance" category (table 5.3).

It's a refreshing change from herpes and HPV, which come with so much more baggage. The worse news is that it is time to talk about the most serious STDs, which have the potential to be life threatening and life limiting.

CHAPTER 6

# Treatable, Incurable, Potentially Life-Limiting STDs

Sex can be a germ spill,
People aren't safe for real

I WAS ASKED to lead a discussion with the older women's Bible study at my downtown church because a few of the women had heard of my rap video about STDs ("STDs Never Get Old"), and they were curious. I was told that this group of 20 or so 60-plus-year-old women met once a month to discuss various topics in one of the members' homes, after sharing fellowship and dinner together.

I arrived that evening after a long day in clinic wearing my "STD scrubs." (I wear scrubs to the STD clinic for two practical reasons: one, my husband made it clear that on STD days I am to wear clothes that can promptly go into the wash upon arrival home, and two, statistically speaking, the odds of getting body fluids on yourself is higher than average.) I was tired and regretting that I had committed to this unusual venue and another night away from my family.

Usually, my public speaking is in an auditorium or an online venue, and I have grown to prefer large groups simply from a time-management point of view. I like to project my presentation on a large screen because, as entertaining as my stories may be, nothing beats a good picture combined with the backstory. I knew this would be different. The church secretary informed me that there would be no screen or projector, just a living room and attentive faces.

The living room was spacious but not designed to accommodate audiovisual equipment, so the computer and projector I had brought along would be of no use. I rationalized that it was just as well—surely these women had seen their share of genitals in their lifetime and didn't need the classic pictures of pus dripping off the end of a penis or anal warts to help tell the story. Since I was not sure how this would roll out, I had done some homework and had filled up several 2-foot by 3-foot sticky-note papers with fill-in-the-blank questions, true/false statements, anatomic drawings with lines to label, and discussion questions. As I prepared this the evening before, I'd prayed that I wouldn't horrify, bore, or overwhelm these aged ladies with this incredibly nontraditional Bible study content.

I was greeted with incredible enthusiasm and kindness as I made my way around the room, meeting the various attendees. I am fairly certain the average age was well above 60. After a lovely covered-dish dinner, everyone gathered in the living room with my big sticky-note presentation front and center.

What followed was the most energetic, honest, and riotous two hours of my STD teaching career. The women were surprisingly eager to learn.

"I don't understand, you can do *what*?"

"I can't even imagine such a thing!"

"Oh, yes, that's very good advice."

"I have a friend . . ."

These women were not afraid to ask tough questions, to be open about their concerns about friends, and to try to understand a reality for their grandchildren very different from what most of them had lived. By the end of the night, all the ladies were text messaging either their grandchildren (if they were teens or young adults) or friends, encouraging them to get the HPV vaccine, to use condoms, to make sure they were getting tested. Their enthusiasm was . . . infectious!

The ladies were particularly alarmed to learn about, and understand more fully, the link to cancers from HPV and the many life-threatening STDs that are out there. This chapter focuses on some of the most common sexually transmitted infections and the ones older adults will surely encounter. In many ways, it is the scariest because the infections in this chapter have a significant risk of being life-limiting or leading directly to death. While it is possible to die from syphilis, unless you are an unborn or newborn baby with congenital syphilis, it is highly unlikely in our advanced state of medicine. The rare herpes encephalitis I spoke of in chapter 5, which can occur when the first herpes outbreak spreads to the brain, can be deadly, but the odds of that happening are really quite small. And while I have had patients who said they would die when I told them they had genital warts, the evidence points to the contrary.

Unfortunately, statistics tell the story of new HIV (human immunodeficiency virus) and hepatitis C infections in the older demographic, so it remains important to include this in our time together. In 2012, the Centers for Disease Control and Prevention published a *Morbidity and Mortality Weekly Report* saying, "More than 2 million U.S. baby boomers are infected with hepatitis C—accounting for more than 75% of all American adults living with the virus." But hepatitis is only one of the many diseases threatening the older community. The CDC reported that in 2016, nearly half of the people in the United States living with HIV were aged 50 and older. In 2017, one in six new HIV diagnoses were people over the age of 55, and in 2018 there were 37,968 new HIV diagnoses in the United States, with 17% of these in people aged 50 and older. Older patients represent the largest increase in treatments of STDs seen by health care providers' offices.

## HIV/AIDS

It was 1988. I was a junior in high school and part of an elite theater group in our city that was audition-only, with participants from high schools all over the county. Our director, Dan "Sea" Seaman, had written an incredible ensemble production with his students two years prior called "The Whispered Word" about teen suicide. It went on to win numerous competitions and was transformative for many adolescents. Early in the fall semester, gathered in the polyester orange seats of the Weaver School theater, we were buzzing with excitement. Sea had just shared that we would be going on a trip to Washington, DC, to do research for a one-act ensemble play we would be writing about the "new" AIDS epidemic to take to competition. There was something called an "AIDS Quilt" that would be on display in front of the White House, and we would be writing a play inspired by what we learned that weekend.

In 1988, not many of us were tuned into AIDS, but we had all been awed by "The Whispered Word," and the idea of writing our own one-act to take to state competition was incredible news. Completely unprepared for what we would experience, we had a chartered bus for the trip. It was an amazing weekend, with our first night spent seeing a traveling company perform *Les Misérables*. Interestingly, this first glimpse of Broadway-level theater launched a lifelong gathering of *Les Mis* productions wherever I travel, and frequent singing of *Les Mis* songs at the top of my lungs. It is a rite of passage in my nuclear family that when the kids get old enough to appreciate it, they attend a trip with Mom to see a Broadway production of *Les Mis*.

On the second day of the trip, the bus driver dropped us off in front of the White House, and we walked to the Ellipse on the south end of the National Mall. Our assignment was to find the panel whose story we were going to tell—which character we were going to be—in the play we would write. In front of us, spread out across what would cover football fields, was panel after panel, each 2 feet by 3 feet in size, almost 10,000 in total, each representing someone who had died from AIDS.

We spent the better part of a day walking between the rows, kneeling to read the letters affixed to the panels, viewing the pictures, and sitting with mourners weeping over their loved ones' panels. We were all looking for the one we would honor. I chose David. I think I chose him because he was a father and I could imagine what his children had gone through, losing a dad to AIDS at a time when it was deeply stigmatized and seen as shameful. I was sad for David, a young man, leaving his children to grow up without their father. His panel had a bright sun that resonated with me. In the play, David became my father who was dying of AIDS. The weekend was illuminating—eye-opening—and what can only be described as transformative. I am certain it had an influence on my career. How could I provide a safe haven for those suffering from illness and disease, where they might otherwise feel judged and alone? The AIDS epidemic followed me to medical school.

In the mid-1990s I started medical school, where I learned the true extent of just how deadly AIDS was. The number one cause of death in young people in the early 1990s was AIDS. While the first antiretroviral drug to combat AIDS (a treatment to slow the progression, not a cure) had been discovered in the late 1980s, it was incredibly expensive and not available to everyone. If you did not have health insurance or if your insurance had a high deductible, it was simply impossible to pay for this life-extending treatment. As the virus rapidly developed resistance, the first combination drug was developed; it was made up of two medications, which was much more effective. This was only released the year I started medical school, meaning that we were still admitting patients—mostly young, beautiful men—in advanced stages of AIDS. Their rooms were isolated with big barriers outside the door and obvious signals to the staff to gown up prior to entering. The negative stigma attached to AIDs was brutal and quite astonishing. There were so many misconceptions around how you could and couldn't contract the disease that people were afraid to go near AIDS patients. You might remember Princess Diana making international headlines when she hugged a young Black child in the AIDS unit of a New York hospital while on a tour. Their deaths were painful and often gruesome as their bodies were consumed by infections and cancers like Kaposi's sarcoma (a cancer that causes disfiguring purple lesions on the skin and lymph nodes). Everything about AIDS was heartbreaking.

Luckily, in the several decades since, health care providers have become so adept at treating HIV infection that we rarely encounter an AIDS death, and most people with HIV infection die of other causes. The federal government subsidizes the provision of HIV medications, so the financial barriers that kept people from treatment in the 1990s have not persisted. However, just because you are less likely to die from HIV does not mean living with it is easy. The treatment is a drug cocktail that requires frequent dosing multiple times a day and carries with it significant side effects, including nausea and vomiting, kidney and liver damage, and the development of diabetes and heart disease.

We have been so effective, in fact, at the management of HIV infection that most people on the drug regimen will actually live for years with no virus detectable in their blood. Why is that significant? We have learned that if the virus is sufficiently suppressed, it cannot be transmitted to others. "Whaaaaaaat?" you might be asking. Yes! The phrase "Undetectable = Untransmittable" is now widely used to help break down the stigma of HIV infection.

With the advent of hookup apps, there has recently been a steady increase in HIV infections, often with co-infection with hepatitis C or syphilis. HIV is an infection of the young and the old. In 2018, the CDC estimated that almost 400,000 of the 1.2 million people living in the United States with HIV were over 55 years of age. And while 9 in

10 of those people knew they had the infection, 1 of them did not. Could you be that person?

Many of the people infected with HIV in the late 1990s and early 2000s survived thanks to the first rounds of successful treatment and are now in their 50s, 60s, and 70s. This means that statistically, the chances of a new partner having HIV could be significant. The CDC provides reassuring data that those over 55 living with HIV are more likely to adequately suppress the virus with medications, but that is still only 64% of those infected, leaving 36% not virally suppressed and infectious. Older adults are less likely to have regular testing and more likely to present with a new HIV infection at a more advanced stage, where the impact to the immune system is more significant.

It's not all dismay and despair though. There is also a relatively new option available for anyone engaging in high-risk sex. It is a daily medicine referred to as PrEP (pre-exposure prophylaxis) to prevent acquiring an HIV infection from having unprotected sex. Who might benefit from PrEP? A colleague shared a story of a patient of hers who had lived a very peaceful, monogamous married life and raised a family, but after his wife of over 50 years passed away, he finally felt able to honor his true desires. He began dating men and became very active, having unprotected sex with multiple male partners often identified through hookup apps. This made him a great candidate for PrEP. Anyone who is switching between male and female partners, who has multiple partners, or who is not reliably using a barrier method should consider taking PrEP. Finally, anyone who trades sex for drugs or money, or uses IV drugs and shares needles, is a great candidate for PrEP as well. Maybe when you are reading this, you are not thinking of yourself but of someone else in your life who might benefit from this potentially lifesaving and life-changing drug.

Getting started on PrEP is incredibly easy. Insurance covers the cost. It just requires some lab work to be certain your kidneys and liver are healthy enough and to ensure that there are no possible

TABLE 6.1. Basics of HIV

| Cause of Infection | Human immunodeficiency virus (HIV) |
|---|---|
| Type of Infection | Virus |
| Symptoms? | Acute illness with infection then asymptomatic until disease progression |
| Duration of Infection | Lifetime |
| What It Can Infect | Most typically mucosal entry point or through shared needles |
| Preferred Test | Saliva, blood NAAT |
| Test Time to Results | Immediate (saliva), 24–48 hours (blood) |
| Insurance | Broadly covers |
| Treatment | Antiviral drug cocktail |
| Partner Treatment? | Yes, if positive |
| Reportable? | Yes |
| Typically Found | Most common in men who have sex with men |

drug interactions. As long as your screening labs are negative for active HIV, and your kidney and drug check are clear, it's a great option to prevent getting infected with HIV. Regardless of what you think your risk is and whether or not you might benefit from PrEP, sexually active adults should have an HIV screening test every year (table 6.1).

## Hepatitis B and C

"Hepatitis" means inflammation of the liver, and it can be caused by a variety of factors such as infection, toxic exposures, and autoimmune disease. Hepatitis can lead to liver failure, liver cancer, and death. While some treatments are available, many people with chronic infection are unaware they have the disease while it is slowly damaging their liver. Common things like taking acetaminophen (Tylenol) and drinking alcohol (beer, wine, liquor) can further worsen the damage to the liver. There are several specific viral infections (creatively named A, B, C, D, and E) that can cause hepatitis, and two of them (hepatitis B and C) fall into the category of being sexually transmitted. Both can also be transmitted by blood, and in fact, for many years we did not know hepatitis C could be sexually transmitted. I am going to cover them together in this section for the sake of simplicity, although with advances in pharmaceuticals in the past decade, hepatitis C officially falls under the category of "Treatable and Curable." However, because it is so often overlooked and undiagnosed, it has led—and continues to lead—to a large number of deaths. The CDC reported in 2016 that hepatitis C was the cause of the highest number of deaths in the United States due to any single infection, with the greatest burden falling on the baby boomers, according to Healio, an infectious disease news source.

> "Land ho!"
> It's a tsunami! Acute hepatitis B!
> Preventable with vaccines, you see.
> Drug users high risk—
> Risky sex (tsk, tsk)
> Should be vaccinated, why not? It's free!

I will tell you the story of Ray, who was almost 55 and died a tragic death from hepatitis C and alcoholism. He had been infected with hepatitis C several decades earlier, during a self-described "wild time" in his youth when drugs ran his life. Ray was a quiet man who lived with the shame of a lifetime of bad decisions, and regret was always painted across his face. He was embarrassed by his history of IV drug abuse and did not like to talk about it, even when I assured him that he had survived and conquered that addiction, making him stronger than he was giving himself credit for. While he had been able to put aside the drugs, he was a slave to alcohol and would drink a case or two of beer daily and more on the weekends. The combination of his untreated hepatitis C infection and daily alcohol consumption meant Ray was dying prematurely, well before he should have.

He was uninsured and had never qualified for disability despite our many efforts, including hiring a lawyer to help him appeal the decision. I wrote passionate letters outlining why he would never be able to meaningfully work at this critical juncture due to his failing health, but they went unheeded. In the five years that I cared for him, he was never a candidate for what is now "the old" hepatitis C treatment, Interferon (which was still relatively new then) for three reasons: (1) he could not afford it, (2) he was still drinking alcohol daily, and (3) he suffered from severe bipolar disorder. The early treatments for hepatitis C were crushing for those with mental illness, and this made him a terrible candidate—even if he could have afforded it or a specialist had been willing to take him on for free. These same challenges made him a terrible transplant candidate, so he never made the transplant list for his liver failure.

I saw Ray in the office a lot, sometimes daily, when in the throes of liver failure because of alcohol consumption, and sometimes monthly, when he would periodically dry out. When he would relapse, he would come into the office confused and trembling, his brain swollen by the toxins his liver was unable to process. We would frantically tweak his medications to try to pull him out of it and bring him back to a coherent and lucid state. We insisted on daily visits to determine if he needed hospitalization, until Ray could no longer manage the ravaging side effects of hepatitis on his own from home.

The last time I saw Ray was only hours before he died. I had come to do a "social visit" in the intensive care unit (ICU). I was sitting on the side of his hospital bed, holding his hand and telling him there was nothing left that could be done. I had come to say goodbye. His liver failure was the worst it had ever been, and he was in the ICU, bleeding internally. We had talked about this day coming for years. He knew his ongoing drinking was leading to his death. But as I sat on the side of his bed that day, he told me he wasn't ready to die. He cried then, and I cried with him. The unnecessary deaths of people like Ray could be avoided with the expansion of health care to all people; unfortunately, he fell through the very large cracks that are common in our health care system. As other states have expanded Medicaid, the cracks have gotten smaller, but at the time of printing this book 13 states have still failed to extend coverage, and people continue to suffer and die prematurely from lack of access to affordable health care. Ray and the many patients like Ray whom I have sat with in their final moments have left an imprint on my heart that motivates me to try to change our system for the better.

If Ray had lived another few years, he would have qualified for the new hepatitis C treatment, which can be given without difficulties to patients with mental illness. As opposed to Interferon treatment, which caused severe depression and suicidality, the newer drugs have none of those side effects. If Ray had been able to qualify for disability or Medicaid, he would have been able to access a higher level of treatment for addiction and mental illness. Instead, Ray died at age 55 with the bleep of the monitors as his only companion.

A treatment and cure for hepatitis C was discovered in 2013, but it has not yet turned the tide of this infection's impact on the population of the United States. A 2019 blog post from Health in Aging summarized recent research on the treatment of hepatitis C: "A hepatitis C infection can be particularly serious for older adults, since many don't seek treatment until the condition is in advanced stages. What's more, hepatitis C is considered harder to treat for older people who have lived with the condition for a long time compared to younger people." The article the blog references contains research that shows that even though older adults are more likely to have advanced disease, they can also have excellent results with the newer treatments now available.

With well over 2 million Americans living with hepatitis C infection, if you have not been screened for this before (with a simple blood test), you probably should be. Because hepatitis C was present in blood products for transfusions and was not tested for routinely in transplant patients until 1992, many people harbor a silent, chronic infection. Over half of the people who become infected develop a chronic infection, and many of the people in the United States living with hepatitis are unaware of their infections. The US Department of Health & Human Services states that 67% of people with hepatitis B and 51% with hepatitis C are unaware they are infected.

The current recommendations are that all adults aged 18–79 should have a one-time screen for hepatitis C, as it often creates an indolent infection that goes years or even decades without causing any symptoms. It results in many deaths in the United States, where it is the number one cause of liver transplants. This screening identifies an old infection, so if people are engaging in high-risk unprotected sex, they should get tested every year.

While there is not a vaccine for hepatitis C, hepatitis B solidly falls in the category of 100% preventable. According to the Hepatitis B Foundation, "Two billion people (or 1 in 3) have been infected and about 300 million people are living with a chronic hepatitis B infection. Each year up to 1 million people die from hepatitis B despite the fact that it is preventable and treatable."

Yes, you read that right: It's totally preventable with a readily available vaccine. Hepatitis B is transmitted through blood and body fluids, like hepatitis C, and it is the number one cause worldwide of liver disease and the leading cause of liver cancer. In the United States, it occurs at a lower rate than hepatitis C, which has risen in recent years due to the opioid epidemic and increased use of IV drugs. Unlike hepatitis C, which now can be cured with new antiviral drugs, there is no cure for hepatitis B, although there are treatments that can decrease the inflammation of the liver.

Decades ago, a vaccine was developed that became required in health care workers and routine in children to protect against infection with hepatitis B. Unfortunately, if you are in the demographic this book aims to educate, the odds are good that you have not been vaccinated against hepatitis B. But you may still qualify for the vaccine. Below are the populations that the CDC recommends receive the hepatitis B vaccine series:

- All infants, beginning at birth
- All children aged <19 years who have not been vaccinated previously
- Susceptible sexual partners of hepatitis B–positive persons
- Sexually active persons who are not in a long-term, mutually monogamous relationship (e.g., >1 sex partner during the previous 6 months)
- Persons seeking evaluation or treatment for a sexually transmitted disease
- Men who have sex with men
- Injection drug users
- Susceptible household contacts of hepatitis B–positive persons
- Health care and public safety workers at risk for exposure to blood
- Persons with end-stage renal disease including pre-dialysis, hemodialysis, peritoneal dialysis, and home dialysis patients
- Residents and staff of facilities for developmentally disabled persons
- Travelers to and families adopting from countries where hepatitis B is common (e.g., in Asia, Africa, South America, Pacific Islands, Eastern Europe, and the Middle East)
- Persons with chronic liver disease, other than hepatitis B (e.g., cirrhosis, fatty liver disease)
- Persons with hepatitis C infection

TABLE 6.2. Basics of hepatitis B and hepatitis C

| Cause of Infection | Hepatitis (B, C) |
|---|---|
| Type of Infection | Virus |
| Symptoms? | Variable |
| Duration of Infection | Years to lifetime |
| What It Can Infect | Liver |
| Preferred Test | Saliva C, blood B,C |
| Test Time to Results | Saliva C immediate, blood 24–48 hours |
| Insurance | Broadly covers |
| Treatment | Antiviral medication |
| Partner Treatment? | Yes, if positive |
| Reportable? | Yes |
| Typically Found | Increasingly found in men who have sex with men |

- Persons with HIV infection
- Adults with diabetes aged 19 through 59 years (clinicians can decide whether or not to vaccinate their diabetic patients ≥ 60 years)
- All other persons seeking protection from HBV infection—acknowledgment of a specific risk factor is not a requirement for vaccination

We will conclude our very limited discussion about hepatitis with table 6.2 as a quick reference. There are many comprehensive resources on the topic of viral hepatitis, and this infection has the potential to wreak much havoc and is often overlooked by lay audiences for its sexually transmitted nature.

### Human Papillomavirus: Cancer

You have already learned a lot about this tiny ubiquitous virus, human papillomavirus (HPV), in chapter 5 as the cause of genital warts, and you learned about the vaccine to prevent infection. Now it is time to learn about the ways an HPV infection can lead to death.

There is a reason why nuns don't get cervical cancer. A correlation between sexual activity and certain cancers was recognized nearly two hundred years ago, when, in 1842, an Italian physician observed that sex workers were more likely than nuns to develop cancer of the uterus. In fact, unless a nun has a busy life (including sex) prior to entering the convent, they tend not to get HPV-associated cancers (which are almost 100% of cervical cancers), while the rest of society is at risk. Therefore, unless you are a nun or have never had sex in your life, the chances of having "run into" HPV are pretty high, and that means you too may be at risk for an HPV-associated cancer. The graph in figure 6.1 shows the high percentage of adults aged 18–59 with genital HPV infection almost 10 years ago, so some of these same people are now in their late 60s.

The trends of cancers due to HPV are shocking. What is startling about the graph in figure 6.2, which depicts the trends of HPV-associated cancers, is the dotted line, which shows a rise in HPV-associated cancers that are not cervical, while there is a nearly simultaneous decline

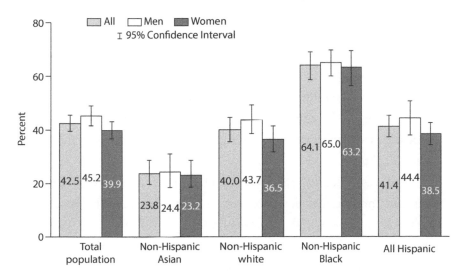

FIGURE 6.1.
During 2013 through 2014, prevalence of any genital human papillomavirus was 42.5% among adults aged 18–59, 45.2% among men and 39.9% among women. *Source:* cdc.gov

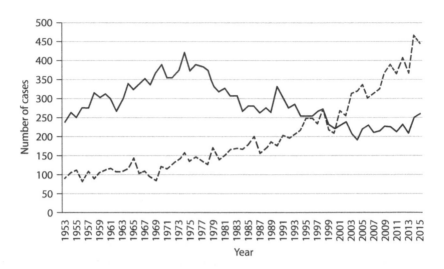

FIGURE 6.2.
Number of incident cases of cervical squamous cell carcinoma (SCC) (solid line)
and all other human papillomavirus (HPV)-related cancer combined (dotted
line) in Norway from 1953 through 2015. Combined cancers: cervical adenocar-
cinoma, vaginal SCC, vulvar SCC, penile SCC, oropharyngeal SCC
(both sexes), anal SCC (both sexes). *Source:* BMJ Journals,
https://bmjopen.bmj.com/content/8/2/e019005

in cervical cancers. The decreased rate of cervical cancers is explained
by the discovery of the "Pap smear," which allows us to screen for cervical cancer and definitively treat women with a precancer or, at the
very least, before it begins spreading. Cervical cancer is almost 100%
associated with infection with HPV, making the Pap smear one of the
oldest STD tests.

Oral, vaginal, and anal sex can all be routes to share HPV infection that can later develop into cancer. With the majority of adults
engaged in oral sex, and an increasing number of men and women
engaging in anal sex, it is not surprising to see the prevalence of the
high-risk subtypes that can cause cancer in so many men and women.
Figure 6.3 shows the prevalence of high-risk HPV in the oral mucosa
of adults.

Remembering that HPV is worsened in patients who smoke or
use tobacco products, I will tell the story of Bob. It was a routine day

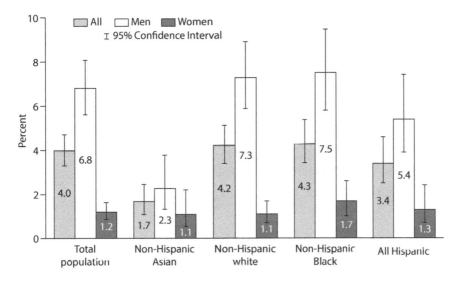

FIGURE 6.3.
Prevalence of high-risk oral human papillomavirus among adults aged 18–69,
by race, Hispanic origin, and sex in the United States from 2011 to 2014.
*Sources:* NCHS, National Health and Nutrition Examination Survey,
2011–2014; cdc.gov

in the walk-in clinic, very busy with lots of flu and strep throat in the kids, and the occasional UTI peppered in. My next patient was a man in his 40s who had a "funny area in his mouth." My deduction game went immediately to a potential list of diagnoses before I entered the room: a syphilitic chancre, thrush, an aphthous ulcer, glossitis, a genital wart.

He was a burly construction worker who avoided health care at all costs. He did not have health insurance and had been trying to ignore the area in his mouth that seemed to be growing for several months. He chewed tobacco and wondered if it was from that, so he had switched sides for several months, but it did not seem to get better and was actually worsening. It did not itch or hurt and was getting larger, despite his efforts to avoid irritation.

He was married and monogamous and drank alcohol on occasion but not with regularity and had no chronic illness that he knew. He had not been to a health care provider or dentist in many years due to the cost. With construction wages not being substantial, combined with the burden of supporting a family of four, health care was the last thing they thought about paying for, unless it was a crisis.

I was immediately concerned when I saw the lesion in his cheek and convinced him he needed to see a specialist for a biopsy, even though I knew how much it would cost. He ultimately agreed and saw an ENT the following week. His biopsy confirmed the presence of high-risk HPV-associated oral cancer.

According to the CDC,

> The median age at diagnosis (the age at which half of cancer patients were older and half were younger) is:
>
> - 49 years for HPV-associated cervical cancer.
> - 68 for HPV-associated vaginal cancer.
> - 66 for HPV-associated vulvar cancer.
> - 69 for HPV-associated penile cancer.
> - 62 among women and 59 among men for HPV-associated anal cancer.
> - 63 among women and 61 among men for HPV-associated oropharyngeal cancers.

What specific body parts are at risk for HPV-associated cancer? The cervix, vulva, vagina, penis, anus, rectum, and throat (including the tongue and tonsils) are all locations of HPV-associated cancers. Increasingly, celebrities have acknowledged they suffered from HPV-associated cancers, including Michael Douglas, Roger Ebert, Marcia Cross, and Farrah Fawcett. Many others died of throat cancer before HPV subtyping was available, and there is speculation that Sigmund Freud, Sammy Davis Jr., and Ulysses Grant all had a pretty good likelihood of having had the infection.

What is the link these people had (besides HPV as the cause of 90% of throat and anal cancers)? Smoking. As I mentioned in the prior chapter, the link between HPV and the use of tobacco products is not clearly understood, but it is repeatedly demonstrated. It is an accelerant to the fire that is HPV-associated cancer.

Switching gears, only slightly, but following this HPV-associated cancer story, let us consider foreskin. Yes, you read that right, foreskin. A great pendulum in health care has been the pros and cons of the newborn circumcision. I recognize that many of you reading this book are not particularly concerned about foreskin right now, and it is not really a "current event" topic for your demographic, but it's an interesting story. The controversy has gone back and forth on whether it is helpful or harmful to circumcise newborn males. The decision is often made in the United States based on cultural and familial norms and not necessarily on science. The most recent data are from studies largely coming out of Africa, which suggest that circumcision has been directly linked to a decrease in both HIV and HPV infection in men, which correlates with—wait for it—a decrease in penile cancer down the road.

With only half of adolescents getting the HPV vaccine series, the risk of penile cancer remains heightened in males who are infected with HPV. Parents are increasingly being asked to make big decisions for their children about future risks they may or may not incur as sexually active adults. Obviously, the question of circumcision comes at birth, but the question of the HPV vaccine, which I have (hopefully) convinced you is monumentally important for everyone who can get it, comes later on in life. While some adult men will have a circumcision due to recurring infections, it is a larger surgery and much more painful as an adult. As grandparents or even great grandparents, I hope you will use your newfound knowledge to help encourage the healthiest possible future generations.

The HPV-associated cancers, HIV, and AIDS make up the most depressing chapter on the STDs, showing that some STDs can be life-threatening and life-limiting. What can you do to avoid these infections? Barrier methods like condoms and dental dams are critical to

TABLE 6.3. Basics of human papillomavirus high-risk subtypes

| | |
|---|---|
| Cause of Infection | Human papillomavirus (HPV), > 100 benign subtypes |
| Type of Infection | Virus |
| Symptoms? | Variable, asymptomatic, warts, invasive cancer |
| Duration of Infection | Lifetime |
| What It Can Infect | Urethra, vagina, cervix, rectum, anus, mouth, tongue, lips, throat |
| Preferred Test | HPV testing on cancer screening/diagnosis only |
| Test Time to Results | N/A |
| Insurance | Broadly covers cervical cancer screening |
| Treatment | Warts: variable, topical home treatment or in-office treatment |
| Partner Treatment? | No |
| Reportable? | No |
| Typically Found | Everywhere, all the time |

prevent infections that can be spread by body fluids, such as HIV, hepatitis B, and hepatitis C. Barriers will help with HPV, but they are not as complete in prevention, and of course, vaccines for hepatitis B and HPV for those who qualify are important! Prevention with regular screening tests is the next most important line of defense (table 6.3).

## CHAPTER 7

# The Great Mimickers: Things That Are Probably *Not* STDs

All these STDs really are stealthy
Without 'em your sex life can be healthy

THIS IS THE CHAPTER you have all been hoping and waiting for. What if you have signs or symptoms of something that is not an STD? Despite my tendency toward assumptions to the contrary, there are many things that can happen to the genital areas that are not sexually transmitted but can make you concerned and decidedly uncomfortable. Most of the conditions on this list are benign, meaning they won't cause cancer or other complications, but some symptoms serve as a sneaking sign of more serious conditions. For that reason, it is always the better side of caution to see your primary care physician (PCP), gynecologist, urologist, dermatologist, or whomever you feel most comfortable with whenever your body changes or looks or feels as though something isn't right.

This begs the question: Do you actually take the time to look at your private parts? This question is not directed at you men. We know you look at your parts. For women, though, the stigma and shame attached to genitals goes back centuries. You may not even know you feel ashamed until you pull out your mirror to look at yourself more closely and are plagued with a creeping sensation that you are doing something wrong. I promise you that you are not. You should be keenly aware of all areas of your body. If you saw a mole on your shin begin to darken and change, you would undoubtedly make an appointment to see your health care provider to get it checked out and likely even biopsied.

Do you know your genitalia well enough to be aware of changes? You should!

Some medical concerns that derive from our private parts and our sexual organs need to be seen and treated by specific and specialized doctors. This is probably not your cardiologist. Why? Because they specialize in the cardiovascular system: the heart. While your heart may have been broken a few dozen times connected to your reproductive organs, genitalia are not these doctors' specialty area. Most family doctors are comfortable with genital concerns. They know when to send you to a specialist. On the other hand, there is more variability among internists and geriatricians. Some prefer to have Pap smears and genital concerns addressed by the gynecologist or urologist. This is a simple question you should feel comfortable asking your primary care doctor or advanced practitioner. While most every community has an STD clinic through public health, some people feel embarrassed going to a health department when they are insured. As someone who has spent a lot of years in a health department, I assure you that the presence or absence of insurance does not matter to us. We see all comers. If you have significant STD concerns and feel more comfortable in a specialized clinic, call your local health department and ask. Many infectious disease (ID) specialists also treat STDs, and while their expertise should be reserved for more complex care than routine screening, you may already have an established ID doc who is comfortable serving that role.

Regardless of which medical specialist you take your genitalia to, it is important to have someone you trust and feel comfortable sharing all the ways you might (or might not) be at risk for infections. But this chapter is not about sexually transmitted infections. It is about some of the other ailments that will make you lose sleep until you know for sure. I will share a high-level overview of some of the most common things I have encountered in my primary care, urgent care, and STD practice to give you a sampling of some of the wild and crazy ways that your body can behave. From a statistical standpoint alone, you are much more likely to have one of these conditions than an STD, so this chapter is well worth your time and will hopefully provide some relief from the stress caused by all the STDs you've already learned about.

## Rashes That Are Probably *Not* STDs

I am pretty sure that there is an entire textbook out there about rashes of the genital area. If there is not, there should be. There are so many skin conditions that happen in this area that there is no way I can do them justice in one chapter, so think about this as a "teaser" for further, more in-depth investigations, should you desire. The blend of keratinized skin (outside skin) and mucosa (inside skin) doubles down on the types of infections and conditions that can develop in this protected area; add to that the relatively warm, humid environment and—voilà—a recipe for disaster is born. Compared to an STD that could be lifelong or life-limiting, most of these ailments would hardly constitute a real disaster, but any issues with your nether regions can feel dire and need to be checked out.

Genital rashes can present a real diagnostic conundrum. The genital anatomy and mucosa simply look different between people. While the general form and function is pretty standard order most of the time, the subtle and not-so-subtle differences between humans can make diagnosis a challenge for even the most experienced clinicians. It is not uncommon to have a "trial and error" approach and ultimately a skin biopsy to obtain a definitive diagnosis. The most important key to diagnosis is often for the physician to really understand what is new and different from what has always been there. A thorough medical history with attention to changes in soaps, lotions, shaving habits, and external exposures are often clues along the way to revealing the problem.

Many of the conditions that occur in the elbows and knees can also affect the genital area. If you have a tendency toward dry skin or eczema, these conditions can crop up in your groin unexpectedly. The same is true for cradle cap (also known as seborrhea dermatitis), which is a buildup of oily plaques on the skin that can affect the scalp, groin, and eyelids. Psoriasis is a skin condition that can cause skin to build up and create scaly, inflamed patches. It can be incredibly challenging to treat, and there is no cure. Like herpes, it can worsen during times of stress. Often when it affects the genitalia, it looks a little different from the scalp, elbows, or knees, which can lead to delayed diagnoses, misdiagnoses, or incomplete treatments that result in unresolved symptoms that linger for years.

The stigma attached to psoriasis is significant and can cause patients great anguish. Many media campaigns have been launched to try to overcome this. The same can be said for herpes. Both conditions can be relentless but, with advances in modern medicine, both can be kept at bay with appropriate treatment. How common is psoriasis? The National Psoriasis Foundation states 8 million Americans have the condition, as much as 2%–3% of the population. As many as 63% of people who experience psoriasis will have a genital occurrence at some point in their lives.

Fungal infections in the genital area are usually caused by two species: candida (yeast) and tinea (jock itch). They are incredibly common causes of rash in the groin for children and adults, men and women, and can be difficult to completely treat. Like the drug resistance we see with gonorrhea and Mgen, many fungal organisms can be resistant to treatment and require repeated treatments. Making things more difficult for your health care provider, patients often try self-treatment with over-the-counter medications for months, so by the time they go to a health care provider's office the "classic" presentation is drastically modified by partial treatments, making it a challenge to accurately diagnosis and treat.

Another skin condition that can be very upsetting for patients is the loss of normal skin pigmentation caused by vitiligo. This is another autoimmune condition where the body destroys its own melanocytes, the cells that cause pigmentation or color. It is usually asymptomatic but can be distressing when normally pink or brown skin turns stark white. While vitiligo is not harmful, it is important to have it checked out and properly diagnosed because some changes in skin color can be a sign of early cancer.

The first order of business with any genital rashes is to get the patient comfortable again. If you develop genital rash or skin changes, don't delay seeking care. Your health care provider will help rule out high-risk conditions like penile or vulvar cancer, which you will recall is often linked to HPV infection. After ruling out ominous diagnoses, your health care provider will provide you with treatment options to improve your quality of life, first, and sexual function, second.

### These Things That Itch Are Probably *Not* Crabs

Wait a minute! We didn't talk about crabs and pubic lice in our STD chapters. How could we leave out the butt of such amazing jokes? I will sneak these little critters into this chapter because they are not so common anymore especially among older adults. Speaking of bad jokes, let me share my very favorite STD joke:

> What's worse than lobsters on your piano?
> Crabs on your organ!

Would you believe I have only seen one case of crabs in my entire 20-plus years in the STD clinic and that was almost 20 years ago? It turns out, the trend of eliminating pubic hair in all forms, which hit in the early 2000s, seems to have coincided with a marked decrease in these genital pests. Pubic lice attach themselves to pubic hair and can have people scratching their nether regions uncontrollably in public because the itch is so profound. They are actually small insects that resemble crabs, hence the nickname, and feed on the body's blood. They are extremely contagious and spread quickly through sexual encounters. If you are one of the many people who shaves or lasers away all of your pubic hair, then you probably never have to worry about dealing with crabs.

It has been an interesting observation over the course of my career to watch the waves of culture change in genital grooming: from the all-natural bushy, to carved-out patterns, to bedazzled, to pierced, to trimmed, to baby-bottom smooth. The natural habitat for crabs has essentially vanished in this country. My bias is that hair has a purpose. Nose hair has a purpose. You might trim unruly hairs, but you wouldn't wax your nostrils. These hairs prevent germs from going into your lungs and killing you. Pubic hair has a similar evolutionary purpose: protect the species-sustaining reproductive organs. As we age, we have less hair everywhere, including the groin. There are fewer places for the crabs to attach to. Consequently, crabs are not really a problem for the older population.

The first and only time I did see and treat crabs was back when I was in my first year of practice after residency. Everything still felt fresh and new, and each day, I would come to work with a blend of excitement and nerves. I wanted to make people better, but what if I missed something? What if I overlooked a serious symptom? What if I didn't know what something was? All the insecurities of a new graduate blossomed in my head and planted themselves daily. Luckily, on that momentous day, the diagnosis was made by a 5-foot-tall feisty grandmother who held her towering 6-foot-plus-tall teenage grandson by his ear as he hunched over. He did not want to be there.

"He's got the crabs!" she announced loudly so everyone in the hallway could hear. She pulled him into the exam room. As if she was afraid that he would dart from her clutch, she swung him around the door jamb and into a chair with the energy of a spring chicken. Securing the door behind her with her foot, she stood with her hands on her hips.

"Show her. Show the doctor your crabs."

"Grandma," he moaned.

"Do it. Drop your drawers. You didn't have any problem droppin' 'em to get these. You can drop 'em here."

Clearly, grandma was not supportive of premarital sex.

"Hi, I'm Dr. Dowler," I reassured him. "I know you don't want to be here, but I have never seen crabs, and I am super-excited. We can take one and look at it under the microscope together!" I gushed. This did not seem to make him feel better.

Junior dropped his drawers, and his pubic hair was littered with little bugs attached to the hair follicles. We plucked one off and looked at it more closely. Its creepy body was filled with blood that it had recently sucked from his warm pubic area. There are bugs that will bite just about anything; the genital area and buttocks are no exception. Sometimes these bites are subtle and the offending critter is not identified, and other times, like with ticks, it is more obvious. Although neither grandma nor grandson were happy to be in an STD clinic, they were lucky that the diagnosis was easily treated with medication.

Speaking of bugs in private areas, when my husband and I were in college, we went to my best friend Susan's family beach house that her grandmother, Nanny, bought in the 1950s. It remains a tiny beach cottage right on the water, which gets closer to the ocean with each hurricane, and was the perfect place to recover after finals. Exhausted from the academic calisthenics we had just completed, we all made a pact to put our watches in a dresser drawer and hang time up for the week.

Our days were filled with playing card games and quarters, throwing frisbees, and napping. The one challenging element about Nanny's cottage was how small it was. It was really, really tiny! There was no hope for privacy, and we were young and randy. One afternoon, Jared and I took our leave and went for a walk across the island over to the sound side. Well, let's just say one thing led to another, and later that night when we were changing for bed, I noticed a black spot on Jared's lily-white bottom.

"What is it?" he asked somewhat frantically, unable to twist his head round enough to see it, though he could feel something was attached.

I examined the critter that was attached to his rear end.

"A tick!" I exclaimed.

I removed it without difficulty, but the amazing, restful beach week ended with an itchy swollen butt cheek, followed by a bout of Rocky Mountain spotted fever. Tick 1, Jared 0. (Even though Jared didn't directly get an infection from sex, it probably qualified as a sexually acquired infection.) While Rocky Mountain spotted fever is not actually sexually transmitted, there are plenty of creepy crawlers that can bite you with sex outdoors, so stand warned.

Another great "bug on the bottom" story happened a couple of years later. Our best friends in medical school ended up being our next-door neighbors who were easily 20 years our seniors but could out-party us every time. They were founding members of a huge camping party music festival weekend. Several years in a row, we were invited to attend as their honored guests. I always volunteered in the medical tent, which was a motley crew of variably trained good Samaritans. I was a medical student, and it was great experience.

One year, the festival fell in a remote corner of the eastern part of North Carolina where it was flat, dry, and hot, and too far from the ocean to be considered a desirable location. Many of the "younger people" decided to forgo tents and sleep under the stars that week. (By "sleep," I mean assume a position of alcohol-induced unconsciousness.) One such fellow wandered into the medical tent after a nice rest on a bed of flattened pine needles that appeared soft and inviting at four o'clock in the morning. Intoxicated and exhausted from the day's events, he decided to unceremoniously fall to the ground. He was rail thin and was dressed only in sagging shorts and a tank top. He sported bare feet and a scraggly collection of facial hair to accompany a buzzed-cut head. He was coated in red clay dust.

"Dude, hey, yeah . . . Uh . . ." He stammered, unsure where to begin. "So, I think I slept in a nest or, like, something, you know?"

He proceeded to take off his shirt, uncovering dozens—no, hundreds—of ticks affixed to his chest.

It was Alfred Hitchcock–level creepy.

"Holy shit!" I exclaimed, very unhelpfully and unprofessionally. I am much better about uncontrolled expletives these days.

"Dude, that's not the problem area, you know, I can, like, just, like, pick those off," he said. He turned around so I could see his back, which was next-level tick-ridden. The stuff of nightmares.

"Oh my gosh!" I exclaimed, then realized I might be freaking my patient out. "Not a problem," I added quickly. "We can get those off."

"Dude, you think that's something? Look at this! I just can't do these, man, I can't do these myself." He dropped his pants, forming a dust cloud of red clay, and stood buck naked in the medical tent. He was in full view of all who passed, with not a stitch of clothing on. His entire body was riddled with ticks, including his groin. Up and down his scrotum and penis were dozens of ticks, looking more like an ant colony. It was a very long afternoon of gingerly picking little creatures from this poor guy's most sensitive region.

Bug bites are a fairly common occurrence in the genital area, especially for outdoor enthusiasts, and they are generally managed the same way you would a bug bite anywhere else. When things are attached, like ticks, sometimes it helps to have a steady hand and a good angle for removal, but you don't need a doctor for the job. Having said that, if you don't have an extra set of hands nearby that are up for the task, we are happy to help.

Another common itchy area that often assaults the genitals is poison ivy. It is only natural that if you have been pulling vines or chopping logs, or otherwise tearing into an overgrown garden, you will be exposed to some sort of poison plant. Wearing gloves and protective clothing often does the majority of the prevention work. The trick is, when taking off the gloves and garden-soiled clothes, to wash your hands of the invisible oils or they may wreak havoc on unsuspecting skin. If intensive handwashing does not occur, when said person goes to the bathroom, whether to wipe or direct their stream, the oils then take up residence on the genitals, and it festers into a very itching, painful, and uncomfortable situation. It's not a sexually transmitted infection, but it sure will dampen your sex life for a week or two. If your partner happens to be a landscaper, beware. You never know what they may inadvertently bring home.

One of my colleagues shared the story of a patient who came into the clinic with an unusual rash that was blistered, oozing, and horrifically itchy. Both of her breasts were covered, as were her buttocks and her perineum. Was it some bizarre form of herpes? An allergic reaction to a soap or lotion? What in the world could it be? Unrelated to her medical history, the patient happened to mention her new boyfriend was a landscaper and had done great work transforming her yard the weekend prior. Grateful for her newly tamed yard, she thanked her boyfriend with an evening of intimacy that transmitted the stubborn oils that remained even after handwashing, to her most sensitive parts. Unpleasant as it was, it was nothing a round of steroids couldn't fix.

## These Things That Burn Are Probably *Not* Herpes

For as many women and men who have come into the clinic with razor burn or nicked skin from shaving, there are just as many that actually have herpes outbreaks. The challenge with shaving the crotch is that the hair serves an actual purpose: protection. The double whammy of shaving is twofold: the protection is removed, and the act of shaving causes microscopic tears in the skin that are a portal for entry. (Because many infections are shared in the blood, like hepatitis C, it is important for people not to share razors.) Both razor burn and waxing can cause the hair follicles to become inflamed and create red bumps. Sometimes they itch or burn, which can be confusing because the blisters formed by herpes are also red bumps that itch or burn. You can see how one could be mistaken for the other. The trick to knowing the difference is all in knowing your body. Is it a hard red bump, or when you zoom in does it look more like a blister? Is it a tiny cut on the skin, or when you zoom in is it more like an ulcer? Does your "razor burn" always happen in the same place? If so, next time run to the health care provider for a herpes test while it is fresh and has some fluid in it.

Friction burn is also a common problem in the genital area. Whether from masturbating, a different sex position, or a prolonged session without adequate lubrication, it is not uncommon. It's also important to think about what's on your hands when you touch your nether regions.

A young man came into the STD clinic complaining of burning on his penis. The clinician's mind immediately went to "herpes" and asked the nurse to get a viral test kit before she went into the room. She was surprised to discover his skin looked a little red in general, but there were no blisters or bumps or any sign of a herpes outbreak. A thorough sexual history did not reveal any risk factors. No new partners, no high-risk partners. Like many adolescents, he was not generous with details, and she had to work very hard to get his story.

Finally, with the right question, he revealed the burning started while masturbating. Upon further probing, the critical piece of information was unveiled.

"Did you use any kind of lotion or lubricant that was different from normal?"

This is often the culprit.

"No. Uh uh," he said, but then added, "I *was* eating a bag of Flamin' Hot Cheetos though."

Nothing like a little capsaicin and chili powder on the sensitive genitals to warm things up! It's not just chili powder that will make your parts burn. Many of the products on the market to enhance sexual pleasure can be an irritant to sensitive skin. It's a good idea to try a test area before going fully in if you have a tendency to react to topical irritants. One other tip from someone who likes to cook Latin-themed foods and has a family who loves all kinds of peppers—wear gloves when you dice jalapenos and serranos or next time you wipe, you might transfer the oils that didn't come off with normal hand washing. That burning sensation when you pee won't be from anything sexual and may not require a health care provider or treatment, but I'm sure it will burn and could easily have been avoided.

> "Snack Time"
> Who doesn't love cheesy Doritos?
> Or onion dip with some nice Fritos?
> But genitals beware
> To avoid a real scare
> Don't masturbate with Flamin' Hot Cheetos.

There are a few other conditions that cause a burning sensation. Lichens conditions (lichen planus and lichen sclerosis) increase in frequency with aging women (but can also occur in aging men, just less often). These are immune-mediated inflammatory conditions that cause burning and itching. A visual difference in the appearance of the tissue is common with a color change to white (hypopigmentation) and fissures or cracks developing in the affected skin. These are chronic conditions that often require lifelong treatment and have some increased risk for squamous cell cancer, so they should be followed by a gynecologist or dermatologist long term. According to a study done in Germany, the average time from the onset of symptoms to when a person sought treatment was five years.

Complications can be avoided with earlier diagnosis and treatment, so seeking a medical evaluation for genital changes is important. The lichens are not sexually transmitted, but like psoriasis, they can make someone feel very self-conscious about the appearance of their genitalia and cause discomfort with sex. Lichens may not be curable, but they are treatable, so don't suffer in silence. See your health care provider so that you get on the right treatment regimen to put you back in the saddle again!

### These Vaginal Discharges Are Probably *Not* Chlamydia

There are many aspects of being a woman that are uniquely experienced in a way men just cannot understand. The monthly cycle is a prime example. Vaginal discharges are another. Men just don't have an adequate corollary in their bodies to the ecosystem that is the vagina. It is a perfect environment for many things to flourish, with or without their host's consent.

For every young woman in the average clinic with an STD, there are two with vaginal discharge of a non–sexually transmitted nature. Most have tried treatments at home with over-the-counter medications and finally come in when the symptoms become intolerable. All women have vaginal discharge, to some degree. It is a completely normal phenomenon. Like pubic hair, discharge serves a protective purpose: to prevent bacteria from entering the cervix and causing infections. The normal vagina has a slightly acidic pH, which also protects against infection by creating an inhospitable environment for bacteria and viruses. With hormonal changes, like the menstrual cycle and menopause, the pH can fluctuate and create an opportunity for infection. Likewise, introducing outside agents to the vagina with a different pH (douching, semen, vaginal rinses) can modify the balance and create a better environment for bacteria to take hold and cause infections. Just as the visual appearance of genitalia varies from person to person, the nature of vaginal discharge is also unique. It is important for a woman to know what is her "normal," so she can be evaluated when there is a significant change in the color, consistency, or odor of discharge.

As women age, the loss of hormones creates less moisture, and the folds of mucosa become more flattened, thinner, and dry. It's not very different from the skin changes you might see on the rest of the body. Many young and middle-aged women are plagued with recurrent vaginal infections, whereas older women who have traversed the mighty menopause become vulnerable to atrophic vaginitis (the inflammation that comes as a result of the loss of estrogen). The young and the old succumb to yeast infections related to antibiotics or uncontrolled diabetes. But did you know that yeast infections are often caused from sex toys that have not been appropriately cleaned between each use? Men are less likely to have genital yeast infections unless they are uncircumcised. Men who do have yeast infections are often asymptomatic or only have a mild "dry skin" appearance to the penis. Partners can toss the yeast back and forth—keeping the infection persistent—and can even cause thrush or yeast in the throat. While yeast is not formally seen as a sexually transmitted infection, it can be an uncomfortable side effect to sexual intimacy that requires treatment.

There are some things that women can do to reduce their risk of these recurring vaginal infections that cause discharge. Perhaps the most important one is to avoid douching or medicated vaginal rinses unless recommended by your physician. As I mentioned above, these things drastically change the pH of the vagina. Historically, douches were recommended to maintain vaginal cleanliness, but what we have learned is they actually create bigger problems. Feminine rinses can be very appealing for women though, especially after a menstrual cycle, as it helps them feel refreshed and clean, but they actually wipe out the healthy balance of the vaginal flora and allow some bacteria to predominate. This can lead to recurring bouts of bacterial vaginosis, which requires antibiotics to treat.

While in many ways I support the provision of treatments over the counter to add convenience to people's busy lives, they often do not save money. People will often try a selection of products before finally relenting and making an appointment with their health care provider. The broadening market of over-the-counter cures and quick fixes for genital infections creates missed opportunities for health care providers to accurately diagnose a condition. It is becoming an increasing challenge for physicians. The prevalence of asymptomatic chlamydia or gonorrhea infections being misdiagnosed by people assuming they know the cause of their issue means that "self-treatment" (which is incorrect treatment) often delays a diagnosis because the signs and symptoms were muted or masked. As the market produces more reliable at-home tests, and insurance companies agree to pay for them, we will mitigate this problem. But for now, here is the bottom line: If you have a vaginal discharge that is not your body's normal, then get it checked out by your PCP or gynecologist.

## These Bumps Are Probably *Not* Genital Warts

Every now and then someone schedules an appointment in the clinic, and when they get there, they sit in the exam room sweating, eyes wide in panic. These are not the same people with a hypochondriac-like obsession with STDs that I mention in another chapter. These people really have something there, but what is interesting is that so often what they are there for is not new; after years of wondering if they were normal, they decide to google their "bumps" and become convinced they have HPV. Even though the bump has been present and unchanged for as long as they can remember, they are worried and decide that it's time for a professional opinion. Their bodies visibly show the relief they feel when I'm able to give them the news that I am not concerned. It is a highlight of my clinical day when I can relay good news to a patient and significantly decrease their stress levels. Our bodies sometime make "bumps" that are not sexually transmitted but are just our normal anatomy. My favorite is pearly penile papules.

Pearly penile papules, also known by the names papillomatosis corona penis, corona capillitii, hirsuties coronae glandis, papillae coronis glandis, and hirsutoid papillomas, are a completely benign finding. They are not sexually transmitted. They are not premalignant. They are not symptomatic. They are not related to poor hygiene. They are normal. They are small bumps that occur around the head of the male penis in the "sulcus" region and are small, smooth bumps (not the rough texture like warts or the umbilicated lesion of molluscum). They develop in adolescence and persist into adulthood but tend to "involute" or fade with advancing age. However, they can be a cause for great alarm and even embarrassment, so some men will seek treatment for cosmetic reasons. If you have bumps that are essentially unchanged and have been present prior to being sexually active, you can probably rest assured that it's nothing to be concerned about. But when in doubt, check it out!

Because so many bumps are in fact related to infection, and some infections can go on to cause cancer, it is the best course of action to have your bumps checked out by a professional. Once you get the "all clear," then go about your merry way, enjoying sexual escapades to your heart's content, but until then, it's best to delay sex and risk sharing something with a partner!

"Things That Go Bump in the Night"
Bottom bumps number so many
But now I will give you the skinny
Until you are sure
And know for sure what's in store
Don't have sex and I *mean*, don't have any!

## The Bottom Line

Many people, when faced with changes in their genitalia, retreat into fear. They will go weeks, months, or even years without seeing their health care provider because they are too embarrassed to ask or are afraid something terrible is happening. Some never look at or touch their genitalia. Some will continue to have active sex lives, while others will hide their genitalia from everyone. Regardless of which person you are, here is my advice: More often than not, there is a reasonable explanation that does not result in great drama and can be managed with medical or pharmaceutical intervention. Rather than obsessively searching the Internet, assuming the worst, inaccurately self-diagnosing, ordering random treatments online, or spending a gazillion dollars on over-the-counter treatments, try making an appointment and asking your health care provider.

While there are more things out there that are not sexually transmitted, it can often be hard to tell the difference. Sex can be messy. Genitals can be messy. Embrace your genitals the same way you would any other body part, and don't ever be embarrassed to talk to your health care provider about them. On that note, let's talk about how we can all do a little better in this area next.

## CHAPTER 8

# Staying on Top of Things (So to Speak)

Wait 'til they're checked at an STD shop,
Check things out from the bottom to the top!

BENJI GRUDGINGLY WALKED into the clinic at the end of the day. He was over an hour late for his appointment and was hoping he would be turned away. He was a "contact" (meaning that he had been exposed) to syphilis and was scheduled to get tested and receive a shot of penicillin (the recommended course of treatment). He had tried very hard to avoid this encounter. Being "a contact to syphilis" means someone named him to the disease control specialist as having been a recent sex partner. His roommate (whom he had recently slept with) had been diagnosed and treated. The disease control specialist had called, left voicemails, sent text messages, and finally waited near the home for Benji to return to force a conversation. These disease control specialists are good! Benji adamantly denied having had sex with his male roommate, but eventually, after the threat of escalating to the health director for an order to report to the county, he agreed to keep an appointment to be tested and treated the next day at clinic. He finally arrived just as we were getting ready to close for the day.

Our disease control nurse, Beth, was an expert on checking for syphilis. She loved STDs almost as much as me. She came in and asked if we would still see him since he was so late. The generally accepted answer was "no" in this particular clinic, but she knew how hard this guy had been to lasso.

"Of course," I said. "But I want to see him. Not just labs and penicillin. A doctor visit too." Originally, he only agreed to blood work and had declined a doctor visit.

With a twinkle in her eye she said, "Sure thing, doc!"

A few minutes later, she returned and leaned against the door jamb to my office. "Welllll," she drawled dramatically, "He is in room 7, but you'd better hurry; he's a runner."

A "runner" is someone who is likely to leave "against medical advice" or even without seeing the doctor. Runners always have something going on that means they really *need* to see the doctor.

Beth shared that he was incredibly anxious, and he continued to deny any sexual contact with the infected roommate or any male for that matter. Curious. Was he too embarrassed to admit to having had a homosexual encounter, or could he be telling the truth? Beth and I pondered this unusual situation together. Why would the roommate name him as a contact? What could be his motivation? Was he mad at him for some housing dispute and thought this would be a good way to get back at him? Had the disease control specialist simply misunderstood? Young men rarely hesitate to share their sexuality these days (which was quite different in the terrifying AIDS era). Benji told Beth, in slightly broken English, that he felt fine and had no symptoms. He did not need to see a doctor but if it was free, he would.

We had a good conversation about his origins and how he came to be in the United States for school. He shared that his home country did not tolerate homosexuality. Because Benji was in the country on a school visa, he was terrified of being sent back home. "When I go home," he explained tearfully, "I will have to marry a woman and live a life that I do not want. I cannot be sent home."

Even after establishing rapport, he continued to deny having contact with the roommate and denied any symptoms of infection at all.

While he had not overtly stated that he had engaged in sex with men, it was implicit in our conversation. He finally consented to let me examine him while he waited for the rapid syphilis test result.

His exam told a story that did not require the test results to know he needed treatment. Immediately, when looking in his mouth, I noticed a large ulcer on the inside of his right lip.

"Benji, does this hurt?"

He shook his head, "I have been stressed and smoke a lot," he explained. "I think I irritate." Like his lip, the entire back of his throat was covered in an intricate pattern of painless ulceration as far as the eye could see. I knew I would have to tread carefully. He was definitely a runner.

"Well, since you have these spots in your mouth," I said calmly, "Why don't I just take a look around and make sure nothing else is going on?"

I grabbed Beth from the hallway to chaperone the exam.

His visual rectal exam revealed well over a dozen anal warts that were inflamed, some of them with dried blood dotting the rough surface. (Remember the young man who passed out when he saw the picture of anal warts? It was that kind of infection.) A digital rectal exam (where the health care provider puts a finger inside) confirmed the presence of extensive warts internally as well. I asked if he had noticed the bumps, and he said he had not really paid attention, but he had noticed spots of blood on the toilet paper after bowel movements at times.

I explained that he had syphilis in his mouth and throat and that he also had HPV rectally and that both were sexually transmitted infections.

He swallowed. "Will they send me back?" he asked with a tremor in his voice.

"No, not at all; it means that you have some infections we need to treat. It means you need to use protection when you have sex. You have to be more careful. And we need to just check for everything today, okay? No one is sending you home," I reassured him.

Beth patted his arm and stayed in the room to talk to him about the shot he would get and, in her kind and motherly way, helped him feel safe in the foreign environment.

The rest of his tests returned the next day. In addition to syphilis and HPV, which we diagnosed on exam, Benji had both rectal gonorrhea and chlamydia in his throat, both without symptoms. He was a bouquet of STDs. Only by the grace of God was his HIV test negative.

Benji could not be truthful with me that day and avoided health care out of fear. Despite having several STDs, which had to be uncomfortable, he was bound to silence and inaction. He did not have a prior reason to trust health care, he was a guest from another country, and he was terrified of deportation. In addition, he was deeply ashamed of his sexual orientation. Being gay could be a death sentence at home. Many factors contributed to his denial of risk and avoidance of treatment. Everyone has their reasons for avoiding health care providers or sharing only part of their truths, but in the long run, it never pays off.

When patients leave out critical information, we run the risk of missing the real problem entirely. In a very busy office, where the sole focus is not STDs, it is easy to imagine Benji's visit totaling a quick question about risky sex, which he would deny, and being dismissed as not at risk. In Benji's case, this would have resulted in the patient (and all his present and future partners) ultimately failing to have testing, diagnosis, and treatment and the progression to a much more serious disease. What a tangled web we weave.

Sexual encounters don't happen in a vacuum. It takes two to tango, and sometimes a bonus person or two is thrown in. Every person who is sexually active needs to be responsible for maintaining proper sexual health, not only for themselves but for their current and future partners. You should not let fear of the repercussions paralyze you—though in Benji's case, his fear was founded on a rational perceived risk to his way of life.

You must ask yourself, what role do you play in your sexual health? Are you an active participant? Are you a hyperactive participant tending toward paranoia and hypochondria? Are you ambivalent? Dismissive? Dissociated? This chapter is not about morality or sin or guilt or any of those holdovers from your childhood. This is about you, just you, and how you choose to take care of your body and allow others to care for you as well.

The reality is that health care in the United States is not ideal. We spend more than any other developed county, and our outcomes are worse than most. The Centers for Medicare & Medicaid Services report states, "U.S. health care spending grew 4.6 percent in 2019, reaching $3.8 trillion or $11,582 per person. As a share of the nation's Gross Domestic Product, health spending accounted for 17.7 percent."

We leave millions of people without access to health care, and those who have insurance often have copays that break the piggy bank. Even with the improvements from the Affordable Care Act, many people have high-deductible plans and delay care. Even if you are well insured and have Medicare and a secondary supplement, health care is still not ideal. With more and more health care providers employed by high-cost health systems, productivity is the driving force, with too many patients scheduled in too little time. Distracted by the heavy documentation requirements to demonstrate our care is not fraudulent, we are often glued to the computer screen checking boxes and clicking fields. Many health care providers do not have the time or take the opportunity to really go to the mat on every aspect of a person's health and social history. This is especially true with sexual health.

According to the National Coalition of STD Directors, "An estimated 19 million new cases of sexually transmitted infections (STIs) occur each year in the United States with an estimated cost of

$12 [billion to] $20 billion (including HIV) in lifetime direct medical costs (in 2006 U.S. dollars)." With staggering numbers like these, it's incredibly important that you take control of your own sexual health and sit in the captain's seat. No one will care about your sexual health as much as you. The first step for you to take control is to understand what the recommendations are for screening for sexually transmitted infections and how they apply to you.

The STI Treatment Guidelines are established by the Centers for Disease Control and Prevention (CDC) and are updated every few years. We have referenced them in several prior chapters. The CDC publishes these guidelines on their website, and they are available to everyone. You paid for these guidelines, as the CDC is a federally funded entity, so you should know and understand them. The CDC has also created a handy smartphone app that is free and great to have at your fingertips. (Next time you see your doctor, ask them if they have downloaded the STI Treatment Guidelines app and, if they haven't, direct them to https://www.cdc.gov/std/tg2015/default .htm.)

The guidelines are straightforward, but they lend themselves to focus on youth and essentially disregard the older demographic. From a statistical standpoint, this makes total sense. When you look at where the vast majority of infections occur and are transmitted, it is decidedly in younger generations. It does create some difficulty for you as you take charge of your own sexual health to be certain you and your health care provider are following the most accurate guidelines. You don't want unnecessary tests, but you also don't want to miss any tests that you should have.

Below are my recommendations for how I would suggest you consider your sexual health screening needs based on low-, medium-, and high-risk categories. Of course, this could change at any moment— these categories, like your sex life, may fluctuate! When you look back at your last year of sexual activity or your last full sexual health screenings, which category best describes your experience?

Low-to-No Risk:
- You do not share body fluids with anyone. (That includes saliva!) In this case, you don't really need to worry about STDs. You do not need screening until you start sharing body fluids.
- You are a woman who has sex with one female long-term partner who does not have other partners (which you hold in near 100% confidence*). In this case, keep up routine maintenance (such as pap smears) for prevention. Pap smears are most likely all you need unless you develop symptoms of infection or discover your partner is exposing you to more risk. Generally speaking, women who have sex with women have the lowest rates of sexually transmitted infections.

Low Risk:
- You have one heterosexual relationship, and your partner has no other partners (which you hold in near 100% confidence*).
- You are a man in a monogamous relationship with a long-term male partner who does not have other partners (which you hold in near 100% confidence*). In this situation, both partners should be screened at the beginning of the sexual relationship, checking in all previously exposed areas of the body (throat, rectum, urethra, blood) and keep up routine preventive care annually. You do not need yearly testing for all STDs unless your relationship status changes, you have concerns about infidelity, or you develop symptoms.

Medium Risk:
- You have had more than one partner in the last year or your one partner has other partners recently or currently.

---

*If you have a doubt, even a shadow of a doubt, ask your health care provider for screening tests every year.

- You use barrier methods most, but not all, of the time with partners, or your one partner does not consistently use barrier methods with other partners. In this instance, you should be tested in all exposed sites (throat, rectum, urethra, vagina, blood) every year, with any partner change and any symptom development.

High Risk:
- You have had multiple partners in the past year.
- You use barrier methods inconsistently.
- You engage in random hookups regularly.
- You are a nonmonogamous man having sex with men or women.
- You are a nonmonogamous woman having sex with men or women.
- You engage in sexual activity with someone who is not monogamous and has other sexual partners—even if you are monogamous and do not take on more than one sexual partner, you are still considered high risk.
- You trade sex for drugs or money.
- In all of these scenarios, you should be tested every 3 months in all exposed sites (throat, rectum, urethra, vagina, blood) and any symptom development.

You may notice that many of these categories require you to have very frank conversations with your partner(s) about their risks. Are they using barrier methods? Are they having other partners or oral, anal, or vaginal sex? What risks are they bringing to the relationship?

I had a comical conversation with my mom on this topic. She is widowed, so there's a very real chance that she could decide to date again. As awkward of a conversation as it may be to have with your own mother, it's a necessary one. She was horrified at the idea of asking someone such personal questions.

"What in the world would you say? How do you begin that kind of a discussion?" she asked incredulously. "You need to write out a script for people to memorize. People aren't going to know how to have those conversations!"

In case you share her abject horror at this kind of dialogue, I will propose a few ways to start a conversation you might have with a partner before you advance your intimacy. The conversation doesn't have to be awkward, stiff, or formal. The more casual and confidant you are when broaching the subject, the more at ease the person on the other end will feel about answering your questions and opening up. You can make it fun and even a little flirty. Here are some examples to consider trying:

- "I really enjoy your company. I'd like to take things to the next level, but before we do, I just want to make sure we're both on the same page. I get tested regularly, and I'm clean. Have you been tested recently?"
- "I know you have dated before me. I haven't been with anyone since my husband/wife died. It makes me a little nervous. How many people you been with in the last year?"
- "Before we move this to the bedroom, it would make me feel a lot more comfortable if I knew a little more about your sexual preferences. I know it may sound weird, but do you mind my asking, do you enjoy the company of both men and women?"
- "I can't wait to take you for a test drive, but I would definitely feel better if you saw your health care provider and had STD testing done before we move things forward. And, honestly, I would feel better if we used some kind of barrier method to keep us safe. Are you comfortable with that?"
- "Before I learn about which sexual positions you like, can you tell me what methods of protection you prefer?"
- "I've dated a few women/men this year, and I'm sure you have too, so it's probably a good idea if we both get ourselves checked

out before we explore each other any further. I promise it'll be worth the wait." (Insert a wink and a smile.)

As unnatural and uncomfortable as it may feel, it is imperative that you have these conversations with potential new partners before you hit the sheets. It's equally as important to be able to talk to your health care provider about your sexual activity. When you go to the health care provider for your STD screening, here's the catch—your screening quality is only as good as your sexual history and the attention your provider is paying to the most recent guidelines. No one should ever feel judged when speaking to their primary care provider about their sexual health. If you do, it is time to change health care providers. I do not want to minimize how awkward the conversation can be. Any health care provider worth her salt should make you feel completely comfortable asking questions and sharing whatever you need to in order to stay healthy. Having said that, why are older adults so poorly tested for STDs? The fault lies with both the health care provider *and* the patient.

### Our Fault

Many times health care providers are at fault. There are a variety of reason why this can happen:

- Your health care provider simply does not ask the right questions or any questions at all about your sex life.
- He/she assumes you are with one partner only or that you are no longer sexually active.
- They gloss over the sexual history and tell you your status, rather than ask, and do not give you a chance to reply and set the record straight.
- Worse yet, they ask a staff person to ask these sensitive questions before they come in the room to see you and do not bring it up again.

- They have not assured you that your health care provider–patient relationship is 100% confidential.
- They may not be well-versed in STDs and don't recognize the symptoms for what they are.
- The health care provider is very formal or uptight and makes you feel judged.
- They run some tests, but do not run all of the STD tests that they should based on your risk factors.

"True Confessions"
Confess! Could you do a little better?
And follow screening recs to the letter?
Hey, call me crazy—
Some docs are lazy—
So screen right and be a trend setter!

Physicians are human too, and sometimes we make mistakes. In order to truly be the best advocate for yourself, you have to be informed and take charge of your health care. Ask questions. Take notes. Make lists. Being equipped with information and armed with the right questions puts you in control of your own sexual health.

An older woman recently shared a story about a time when she felt her doctor judged her. She was in her early 60s and had a Bartholin's abscess, an infection that can occur in a gland in the vulva. She had gone to a doctor who made her feel extremely uncomfortable for asking a perfectly reasonable question. She wasn't sure how long the healing period was. She and her husband enjoyed an active sex life. She wanted to know how long before they could be intimate again so that she didn't have sex too soon and hurt herself.

"My husband wants to know how soon we can have sex again."

She felt distaste in her doctor's reaction, as if her husband was unsympathetic to her medical situation, which wasn't true at all. The doctor's reaction seemed to suggest it would not be normal for her to be interested in resuming sex. Not being a confrontive person, she didn't say anything further. Looking back, she wishes that she had said, "Actually, I would like to know too. I look forward to resuming sexual relations with my husband."

In that instance, this woman felt chastised, as if she was putting up with an insensitive husband. I asked her if she has had other experiences with health care providers minimizing or misunderstanding her questions.

She responded by saying, "I don't ever feel dismissed, but I also don't feel that my yearning for more pleasure in sex gets acknowledged very fully."

Sometimes conversations about sex can feel uncomfortable for a patient to bring up with their health care provider, but once you "break the seal," most of the time you will find the conversation flows, even if you have to initiate it.

According to 2014 study published in the *Journal of the American Medical Association*, adolescents (who have the majority of STDs in this country) had health care providers who failed to take a sexual history in one-third of visits. Even more astonishingly, when they did take a sexual history, the average length of the discussion was 36 seconds. In other words, if health care providers do ask, many of them ask generically and do not investigate the extent of risks and how best to safeguard health. I can't heat up my tea in 36 seconds, much less understand the depths of someone's sexual risks.

I give myriad STD lectures to large audiences of health care providers (family physicians, internists, ob-gyns—you name it!), and the discomfort in the room when we discuss the critical importance of a sexual history is palpable. To be totally honest, I have been guilty of this as well from time to time. As a health care provider, when you have cared for a patient over many years, it is easy to get comfortable and make assumptions. And you know what they say about people who *assume*? You got it. They make an *ass* out of *u* and *me*.

With more and more adults engaging in oral and anal sex, it is more important than ever that we take the time to provide a safe and respectful space for a thorough sexual history (fig. 8.1). A terrific resource for health care providers is an article written by two of my favorite family health care providers, Margot Savoy and David O'Gurek, along with Alexcis Brown-James in 2020, titled "Sexual Health History: Tips and Techniques." Perhaps if your health care provider is not great at having sexual discussions with you, you can recommend it to them. Taking a sexual history is an important part of training for health care providers in medical school, and training will continue in residency, depending on the specialty.

Below are the "5 Ps of Prevention," as taught by the CDC and shown on its website. These tenets of sexual history taking are a sta-

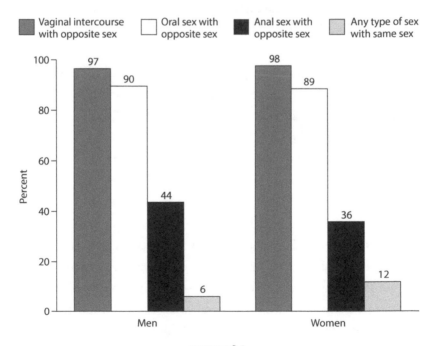

FIGURE 8.1.
Sexual behavior in lifetime among men and women aged 25 to 44 years old in the United States from 2006 to 2008.
*Source:* cdc.gov

ple in a medical student diet today, but it has not always been that way. Providers trained even 25 years ago had a less intense focus on the sexual history. If you feel like your primary care physician, gynecologist, or urologist is not asking you the things they need to ask in order to fully discern your risk factors, you can help them out by giving them some clues.

The Five Ps: Partners, Practices, Prevention of Pregnancy, Protection from STDs, and Past History of STDs

1. Partners
   - "Do you have sex with men, women, or both?"
   - "In the past 2 months, how many partners have you had sex with?"
   - "In the past 12 months, how many partners have you had sex with?"
   - "Is it possible that any of your sex partners in the past 12 months had sex with someone else while they were still in a sexual relationship with you?"
2. Practices
   - "To understand your risks for STDs, I need to understand the kind of sex you have had recently."
   - "Have you had vaginal sex, meaning 'penis in vagina sex'?" If yes, "Do you use condoms: never, sometimes, or always?"
   - "Have you had anal sex, meaning 'penis in rectum/anus sex'?" If yes, "Do you use condoms: never, sometimes, or always?"
   - "Have you had oral sex, meaning 'mouth on penis/vagina'?"
   *For condom answers:*
   - If "never": "Why don't you use condoms?"
   - If "sometimes": "In what situations (or with whom) do you use condoms?"
3. Prevention of pregnancy
   - "What are you doing to prevent pregnancy?"

4. Protection from STDs
   ○ "What do you do to protect yourself from STDs and HIV?"
5. Past history of STDs
   ○ "Have you ever had an STD?"
   ○ "Have any of your partners had an STD?"

   *Additional questions to identify HIV and viral hepatitis risk include:*
   ○ "Have you or any of your partners ever injected drugs?"
   ○ "Have you or any of your partners exchanged money or drugs for sex?"
   ○ "Is there anything else about your sexual practices that I need to know about?"

Interestingly, several organizations are now endorsing a sixth "P" for "Pleasure" and "Pride." For pleasure, it is to investigate whether sexual dysfunction or trauma exists that could benefit from treatment. For pride, it is asking someone about their sexual preferences. These additions are increasingly endorsed by national organizations.

## Your Fault

While sometimes the blame lies squarely with the health care providers, there are plenty of other times when patients have done themselves a disservice by not being fully truthful or forthcoming when asked about their sexual health and risks. Here are some of the ways patients can be to blame for incomplete or inadequate testing:

- You don't tell the health care provider you are in a new relationship since your last screening.
- You don't share what body parts have been exposed to other people's body fluids.
- You minimize your risks in vague terms and allow your health care provider to make assumptions.

- You don't tell your health care provider the full story of how often you use barrier methods.
- You don't *make* your health care provider have the conversation. (Unfortunately, if they are not willing to start the conversation, then you need to take charge of your own sexual health and bring it up.)
- You let your health care provider assume you are in a low-risk heterosexual relationship when you are not.
- You ignore new symptoms and wait them out rather than seeking care.

"Confessions"
STD clinic's more fun when it's juicy—
But I hate HPI* loose-y goose-y.
Most important, I'll say,
At the end of the day,
Is that my patients just tell me the truth-y.

*HPI =History of Present Illness*

Not telling health care providers the whole truth is ubiquitous in exam rooms across the country. In a 2018 JAMA Network article, researchers found that 81% of patients admitted to not disclosing the full story. Why? The number one reason was to avoid feeling judged. If people don't tell their health care providers the truth about a glass of wine, remembering to take pills, or going for a walk, what are the odds people will be comfortable sharing high-risk sex practices?

Part of the problem with talking about sex is just that—talking about it! Generationally speaking, even though the baby boomers were critical to the sexual revolution of the 1960s, there is still a tremendous amount of ingrained teaching about aspects of the body and sexuality as a shameful thing. If older adults had "the talk" with their parents, it was not typically as explicit as conversations today. With teens easily accessing pornography on the Internet, and mainstream television and movies actively addressing sex-related issues affecting teens, talking about sex is not as big of a deal for most young people in this day and age. If you are someone who shies away from open conversation about sex, when you practice saying things out loud alone, you will become increasingly comfortable bringing up previously taboo topics with others.

Remember when I mentioned the sexual health event I convened as part of my Gold Award Project? The most memorable part of that day was the session we did on "Saying No." The subject could easily be viewed as embarrassing for awkward teens who were only still learning about their bodies and sex. But what made it work is that we practiced all the weird and crazy ways you could say, "No" (to sex), out loud to each other. After dozens of repetitions, it became easy to say those words. You can do the same thing with talking about sex if you struggle with this concept.

These exercises are exactly how I teach medical students and residents to become accustomed to taking thorough sexual histories. I give them sexual scenarios and have them role play the doctor–patient sexual history (get your mind out of the gutter—not that kind of role play!). The person playing the "patient" has to stick to the script (with a straight face), which is intentionally graphic and edgy. The examiner has to get the whole story and be impartial, even when the most unusual kinks are described. It is a surprisingly fun lesson. Everyone blushes, most learn about something they have not heard of before, and everyone has practiced asking questions that start off feeling too personal and invasive. Repetition helps to desensitize the interviewer and makes it easier to address these issues with patients.

If you are one of those people who allows your health care provider to make assumptions or gloss over your real risks because you are flustered by the topic of sex, I strongly encourage you to "practice" talking to your health care provider. Do your own role-playing scenarios with a good friend, your significant other, or just your bathroom mirror. The important thing is to say the words out loud, not just in your head. I promise you, it will make it that much easier in the health care provider's office.

Patients and health care providers, alike, benefit from open dialogue. Here are two examples from a colleague and a senior sharing how having open dialogue has been rewarding:

I have been taking care of a 71-year-old man who has been single and celibate for over 30 years, since his wife left him. A few visits ago, he approached me about how to handle sex at his age. He apparently joined an "old people" (his words) dating site and matched with someone. He was terrified because he hadn't had sex in ages. He wasn't jumping to go just yet but was so upset about it happening in the future, he didn't know what to do. We talked about masturbation (he said he was good at that) and how to approach the relationship. We discussed how to spice things up, toys, etc. The main thing we discussed was how he needs to voice his concerns with his partner when he felt comfortable as she may have the same concerns. He had no STDs (yet, lol), but it was a wonderful visit all around.—Dr. Jess

Perhaps having a woman doctor made things easier, but it wasn't awkward to tell her that I was sexually active again at 75, after 15 years of celibacy following the death of my husband of 35 years. She prescribed the necessary treatments for both comfort and the possibility of yeast infections. To find love again, in all its many manifestations, was a predictable joy. What was surprising—and rejuvenating—was realizing that my aging body was physically appealing to my lover, as well as how much his lovemaking aroused me. Freedom from the urgency to bear children on the one hand and the threat of pregnancy on the other makes sex beyond the childbearing years a source of pure pleasure.—Thea, age 79

## A Step Beyond Normal Concern

There is one phenomenon that must be mentioned, even though it is less often encountered in the older demographic. I have dubbed it "the worried penis." The medical name is cypridophobia, which is defined by *Stedman's Medical Dictionary* as having a morbid fear of having an STD or the false belief of having an STD. Over the many years that I worked in migrant health, this was a recurring and frequently encountered circumstance, seemingly triggered by abject guilt following a sexual indiscretion. The negative thoughts would persist for months or even years. Some men would return to the clinic repeatedly, insisting they had "lesions" that no one else could see that needed to be frozen off. After unsuccessfully trying several different providers in the clinic and being denied a procedure to freeze off nonexistent lesions, the frantic patient would demand a urology consult, despite the high medical cost they incurred. Without fail, if I could convince them to be treated with a low-dose SSRI, a type of medicine to treat anxiety and depression, the obsession resolved and their "STD" went away.

> "Oy vey!"
> One of the toughest "STDs," between us,
> Cypridophobia (I call "worried penis")
> Not a speck to behold
> (But they just can't be told)
> This phobia plagues both Mars and Venus!

In all fairness, I have seen women with this same complaint, and they often have a more general bent toward somatization. Somatization is when people manifest symptoms of illness when none are present. Another word commonly used is "psychosomatic," meaning that a health problem only exists in someone's imagination. Differently than men, many women really do suffer from repeated and chronic yeast and bacterial vaginosis infections, which can worsen with the changes of menopause. These women, in fact, have infected genitals. They should not be confused with those who have an unhealthy and obsessive concern about infected genitals.

The treatment of choice for cypridophobia is cognitive behavioral therapy (CBT), a highly effective, evidence-based form of psychotherapy. Let's be honest, everyone can use a little CBT in their lives. However, if CBT fails, or if the patient declines a behavioral health consult, a low-dose SSRI can really change their lives. One unintended benefit of this therapy is that if a man also suffers from premature ejaculation, a side effect of this class of medication can be delayed ejaculation!

## Why Can't We All Just Get Along?

I think we can agree that all of us, both patients and health care providers alike, hold our own parts in the failure to adequately address the sexual health of older adults. It will take all of us working together and committed to excellence to get this right. It will also take a willingness to conquer potentially uncomfortable conversations and come out the other side of them. Like in almost all matters of health care, I am frequently amazed at how often patients do not push us health care providers and the health care system to do better. Why don't we strive for full service when we go to our health care providers?

A few years ago, I was at a ribbon cutting for a new and innovative primary care clinic model designed to advance population health principles. The young, somewhat arrogant, hospital administrator who was speaking (and only knew hospital inpatient operations) compared a primary care doctor's office to a Jiffy Lube—out loud—on the record and in front of the media and several primary care doctors. I was incensed.

Seriously? The cornerstone of the medical home was likened to a Jiffy Lube? I remember looking around the room in complete and utter amazement that such an ignorant metaphor could be cast, but he had moved on. Nobody else seemed bothered. Apparently, I was all alone in my indignation. I see primary care, the medical home, as the crux of a person's health and more of a critical utility than a one-stop convenience.

But, for the sake of progress, let's take that insulting metaphor and apply it to your sexual health. If you took your car to a Jiffy Lube for an oil change, they would ask if you wanted your tires rotated or your windshield wipers replaced, or a variety of other "add-ons" to provide as full (and expensive) a service as possible. If you dropped your car off and, without a word, they only changed your oil, would you be disappointed? Would you wonder why they were missing the opportunity to provide an important service? In fact, if the standard for an oil change included these services and you were not offered them, you might feel cheated and demand it when you returned to pick up your car.

Why is health care so different? Why do so many people hesitate to be assertive or ask questions? It is critical that you advocate for yourself if we (the House of Medicine) fail to provide the opportunity to care for all of you. Now that we have exhausted that topic, let's move on. What else can you do to make sure you enjoy late-life sex and safeguard your body?

## CHAPTER 9

# Playing It Safe: An Ounce of Prevention

Can you really help being sex kittens?
But why can't you wear your little love mittens?

THERE ARE MANY motivations for why you might have picked up this book. Perhaps you are a "sandwich generation" child, and you want to understand the sexual risks your parent(s) might be facing. Perhaps you are a retired widow who has decided it is time to consider the next iteration of love. Maybe you have nothing but time and money, and you are just interested in extracurricular activities! You might just be checking things out "for a friend." Regardless of your motivation, this chapter brings together the many things you have learned about how you can best protect yourself and stay sexually active longer and healthier with a few additional considerations.

Who'd of Thunk It?"
Where there's myth I try to debunk it
As I ride the STD junket
So much can be got!
Nary symptom nor rot.
Folks are shocked, like they wouldn't of thunk it.

I hope I have convinced you that being fully open with your health care provider is critically important to making an accurate and timely diagnosis of asymptomatic (and symptomatic) infections. I hope I have persuaded you that knowing what is "normal" for you means looking and touching your genitalia, so you are aware when there has been a change and can seek care promptly. Along these same lines, going to the health care provider rather than self-treating or suffering for months (or even years) with mild or vague symptoms is also important. What else can you do to protect yourself?

## Barrier Methods

You all remember condoms, right? Perhaps you have even used one before. It turns out that condoms are as old as STDs. According to a gripping historical account in the *Indian Journal of Urology*, the first condoms were described in 3000 BC: King Minos's wife used a sheep bladder to protect her from his semen, which purportedly killed his mistress because it contained "serpents and scorpions." The article takes you from early civilization, through the Renaissance, to rubber vulcanization in the Industrial Revolution. In World War I, the Germans handed out condoms along with ammunition; the Brits and Americans, on the other hand, suffered from an abundance of gonorrhea and syphilis! Interestingly, despite their forward thinking in World War I, Germany made condom use illegal for civilians in 1941 but continued to share them with soldiers, according to an article in the *Hektoen International Journal of Medical Humanities*, which also highlighted a poster used to educate American troops.

Perhaps you used and thought of them more as a pregnancy prevention tool than for preventing STDs back in the day. The good news is, there has been amazing progress in the quality of condoms over time. With the advent of HIV/AIDS, condom use rose exponentially in the late twentieth century. While our seniors are not as good at using condoms, teens and young adults have actually demonstrated patterns of slowly increasing condom use over the past decade. (I like to think all those STD talks have paid off!) According to Planned

Parenthood, over 450 million condoms are sold annually. Now, that is stock I should have invested in! In our marketing-focused society, there is something for everyone: Do you want smaller, bigger, longer, or wider than average sized condoms? Do you prefer colored, flavored, textured, or ultrathin? Even the packaging of condoms has made great progress. Fun patterns, quotes, and designs now accompany your condoms in place of the stodgy old square packet.

Condoms still work reasonably well for preventing pregnancy when used consistently and appropriately, although we have much more effective methods of contraception at our disposal these days (with and without hormones), so I encourage my young premenopausal patients to aim toward long-acting contraception like IUDs or hormonal implants. For the purposes of this book, pregnancy prevention is not on our worry list. For your reading pleasure, think of condoms as the gateway to safe sex. They are not perfect, but they're better than a sharp poke in the eye!

In addition to the good, old-fashioned condoms of yesteryear, today we have a "male" and a "female" condom. Yes, you read that right. A female condom! It is a societal advance in that it allows women to take charge of safe sex if they have a male partner who is not interested or willing to use a condom. In full transparency, it's a little like an inside-out sandwich bag, and I have never met an actual person who used them regularly. I did ask around to a number of my colleagues in the "lady doctor" business. None of them had much to say about the female condom, leaving me to my own devices to wonder about who uses the female condom.

They seem like a great tool for sex workers to protect themselves, except they are expensive (the female condoms, not the sex workers). So perhaps high-class sex workers use them? There must be a market for them because the companies remain in business. I went to Amazon to take my quest for understanding the female condom to the next level. The cost ranged between $11 and $35 per condom. The average was closer to $15 each. That means a female condom costs more than the cost of Viagra, even before it went generic. The male condom price is 50 cents to $1, with plenty of options at 50 cents. So, the female condom is out there, but it costs 30 times more than the male condom.

There is also a barrier method for oral sex performed on women (the equivalent to the condom for men) or for use with oral–anal sex called a "dental dam." This is a thin barrier made of latex or polyure-thane that can be used to cover the genitalia to protect from the exchange of body fluids. These thin sheets, about the size of your hand, come flavored and colored. They are priced more like male condoms, from 30 cents for a very basic version up to $3 each for all the bells and whistles, including colors and flavors. The average is closer to $1.30 each. When oral sex is performed, these decrease the risk of transmission of infection between the mouth and genitalia in both directions. With the increases in HPV-associated oral cancers and the knowledge that oral herpes can infect the genitalia, it is a great option for those who want to be as cautious as possible.

Now you know that in addition to having open dialogue with your partners and health care providers, knowing your body, and seeking care when things are off, using the above barrier methods can protect you from infections that are carried in body fluids. There is still more you can do to enjoy a healthy sex life.

### Choosing (Your Partner) Wisely

In the last decade, the American Board of Internal Medicine Foundation undertook a consumer-facing initiative called Choosing Wisely (https://www.choosingwisely.org). It exists to educate the public on the appropriate use of tests, medications, and interventions based on the evidence for the outcomes. In other words, it provides a check-point for patients to go to when making big or small medical decisions about their health care. Is a procedure or test being recommend based in evidence? If not, what is the motivation? A woman in her 70s

I spoke to who lives in a retirement community said a doctor in her area is offering an expensive "sex procedure" for men and women to "enhance their sex lives," and she was frustrated at her last visit when he seemed more interested in selling her this technology than in addressing her other health concerns. This would be a great opportunity to go to Choosing Wisely and look up a recommended procedure that seems off.

Essentially, by arming themselves with knowledge, people can take control of their health and choose wisely about whether the test their health care provider is suggesting is the right one for them. At the very least, it can be a point for conversation when a costly test is endorsed by a provider that this database says is not recommended based on the evidence. It creates fertile ground for shared decision-making, an increasingly important concept in medicine, particularly with the baby boomers. According to Encompass Health, by 2030 we will have more adults over 65 than children in this country. Baby boomers will dominate our health care delivery system. They have demonstrated that they are educated, engaged, and thoughtful patients looking for a partner in their health care decisions, not a dictator. If you have the option to choose wisely regarding a procedure that is expensive and painful, and the evidence denotes that it will not actually improve your outcome, or you can choose a lesser-known, more time-consuming option that has better outcomes, which would you choose? It is great to make informed decisions about your health.

Think about choosing your sex partners with the same lens. Every partner is not created equally (and, no, that is not a foot size reference). Would you go out and have an invasive, expensive, or painful test without learning more about it? Most would not. The corollary is sex partner selection. Before becoming intimate with a partner, do you understand their sexual history and the status of their sexual health? Are you jumping into something that could alter your life without understanding the risks? Many people don't consider a one-night stand a risk for changing the whole trajectory of their lives, but it can.

For reasons that I try not to take personally, people don't love coming to the STD clinic. It's embarrassing for some. It's stressful for most. At the end of the visit, you rarely leave fully satisfied because there are test results to wait for. Why go through mental pain and suffering unnecessarily for that moment of relief days or weeks later that the test is negative if you could avoid it by choosing your partners wisely? Remember, whomever you are having sex with brings to the bed all the other partners they have ever been with. The most reliable and trustworthy partner should still support routine screening tests.

Sometimes compulsive behaviors are the source of risk taking; this applies to the young and the old. Recently, I saw my clinic schedule had a 72-year-old male with the reason for his visit being "contact to HIV and hepatitis C." I was disheartened. What a tragedy, to have made it to the age of 72 and then have to deal with such aggressive infections and their complicated treatments. It's not a fun way to run the final stretch of the race (particularly when those infections can be 100% prevented with consistent barrier protection).

I opened his chart on the computer and my eyes were immediately drawn to his extensive medication list—over 17 chronic, daily medications. Interesting, I thought. Polypharmacy (having a complex medication regimen) was not the interesting part; rather, it is unusual is to see someone with that many chronic illnesses engaging in high-risk sex. If the person who scheduled his appointment had this right and he was a contact to HIV and hepatitis C, he must have been engaging in high-risk sex.

I was intrigued. This was going to be an interesting visit.

I opened the door of the exam room to find an elderly gentleman who appeared older than his actual years. He was hunched over his cane with his chin resting on his hands and his eyes shut in either slumber or meditation. He was wearing an overstuffed down coat with areas where tufts of stuffing were peeking through holes. His orthopedic-style shoes were wrapped with duct tape at the toes.

"Mr. Smith?" I asked, disturbing his peaceful rest. "I'm Dr. Dowler, and I understand you have some concerns about a possible exposure to HIV and hepatitis C. Tell me more about that."

He was merry and chipper in a slightly disconcerting way. I learned that he was sexually active with males only.

"Any difficulties with erections?" I asked.

He laughed heartily, "Oh no, dear. That part of my life is done. I enjoy oral sex. Giving it. I love giving oral sex!" He repeated.

"Okay, great!" I said, his enthusiasm was contagious. "How many partners have you had in the past three months?"

"Oh, quite a few. I really like oral sex," he said.

Turns out he wasn't kidding. He shared that he performed oral sex on anyone interested in receiving it. This included strangers who were among the city's homeless population. He had one "main" partner, a much younger man in his 30s.

"That's why I'm here, dear," he twinkled. "Matt has problems with drugs. He just tested positive for both HIV and hepatitis C."

I continued to dig into his sexual history to try to understand his risk profile. His "main" partner having HIV and hepatitis C was a major concern, although my patient's only exposure was his mouth, which is much less likely to transmit HIV than more invasive sexual acts like penetrating vaginal or anal sex, according to the CDC. The entirety of his sexual activity was performing oral sex on men.

He wiggled his bushy white eyebrows and said, "You know, I'm very good at it. The secret to success is not having teeth anymore!"

Sometimes it's hard to keep a straight face. This was a very interesting patient indeed! And it got even more fascinating.

"Do you ever trade sex for drugs or money," I asked. I always ask this question because a health care provider should never assume. I have learned that you can't judge a book by its cover in medicine.

"Not drugs. Sex. I pay for sex sometimes," he answered with confidence.

"I'm confused," I said. "You said you only give oral and don't receive oral or anal. What are you paying for?"

He explained that he paid other men so he could give them oral sex—strangers he met at the bus stop sometimes—and he continued to say, even before I could ask, with a vehement, if slightly prim, declaration, "I will never use condoms because I like to taste what I eat."

It can be really hard not to laugh when a patient's honesty is so unabashed. I like my patients to be forthcoming with their sexual experiences, but the commentary that this man added to his responses almost made me laugh out loud. I had to pull the smile from my lips and work to keep my professional face on.

His STD tests were negative that day, but I mentally wrestled with our visit for the days following. When does the natural drive for sex change from being healthy to pathologic to an addiction? Why would a person willingly put themselves at risk on a daily basis, having anonymous unprotected contacts? What motivates someone already flirting with end-of-life health problems to live so close to the edge? His risks would have been 100% mitigated by using a barrier method, and yet he jeopardized it all for the pleasure he received from offering unprotected oral sex. Human behavior is a mysterious thing.

I uncovered an excellent table from the San Francisco City Public Health Department that shows what infections you are at risk for depending on the type of sex you participate in (table 9.1). It is a nice summary of where infections fall depending on where you are exchanging body fluids.

## Kinks, Trauma, and Aging

There are many kinks in the sexual health world. *Kink* used to be formally known as "paraphilic interests" and described unconventional or unusual sexual acts, urges, or desires that were seen as perverted

TABLE 9.1. Know the risks

If your partner is infected, you could get the following STDs:

### By Performing Oral Sex on a Man

Chlamydia

Gonorrhea

Hepatitis A

Herpes

HIV

Shigella

Syphilis

### By Performing Oral Sex on a Woman

Herpes

HPV

### By Receiving Oral Sex: Man

Chlamydia

Gonorrhea

Herpes

Nongonococcal urethritis (NGU)

Syphilis

### By Receiving Oral Sex: Woman

Herpes

### By Anal Sex: Top

Chlamydia

Gonorrhea

Hepatitis B

Herpes

HIV

HPV

NGU

Syphilis

### By Anal Sex: Bottom

Chlamydia

Gonorrhea

(Continued)

TABLE 9.1. (Continued)

| By Anal Sex: Bottom *(continued)* |
| --- |
| Hepatitis B |
| Herpes |
| HIV |
| HPV |
| NGU |
| Syphilis |

| By Vaginal Sex: Man |
| --- |
| Chlamydia |
| Gonorrhea |
| Hepatitis B |
| Herpes |
| HIV |
| HPV |
| NGU |
| Syphilis |
| Trichomonas |

| By Vaginal Sex: Woman |
| --- |
| Chlamydia |
| Gonorrhea |
| Hepatitis B |
| Herpes |
| HIV |
| HPV |
| Syphilis |
| Trichomonas |

| Oral–Anal Sex: |
| --- |
| By Amoebiasis |
| Campylobacter |
| Cryptosporidium |
| Giardia |
| Hepatitis A |
| Salmonella |
| Shigella |

*Source:* Taken from San Francisco City Clinic Website; as we learn more, this list is constantly evolving to include additional infections.

or deviant, but the negative stigma surrounding eccentric sexual behavior has softened. The term *paraphilic interests* is now used to describe behaviors that are pathological, dangerous, or illegal, and the term *kink* is used to describe those who enjoy healthy eroticism and fantasy-based sex play, often incorporating BDSM (bondage, discipline, dominance, submission, sadomasochism). Those who partake in BDSM do so consensually and with clearly defined rules—some even sign mutually agreed-upon contracts. Kinks were found in approximately one in seven people in a study published in 2017 in the *Journal of Sex Research*. Even though relatively common, kinky, out-of-the-box sexual escapades and fetishes are often hidden from health care providers out of shame or fear of judgment. Historically, these sexual preferences have been considered maladaptive or abnormal, but increasingly research suggests that, like many things in medicine, "normal" is actually a broad range that encompasses abnormal at the far end. In many ways, if you are not acting out against someone's will, who is to say what is normal and healthy and what is not? It boils down to moderation versus compulsion. When something becomes all-encompassing and hinders functionality, it borders on a disorder.

The *DSM-V*, the fifth edition of the *Diagnostic and Statistical Manual of Mental Disorders*, developed by the American Psychiatric Association, identifies the most common categories of paraphilic disorders (such as causing pain or impairment), which are differentiated from paraphilia, which describes atypical sexual interests.

- *Voyeuristic disorder:* The erotic interest in watching others having sex, generally without their knowledge. The key element here is that the voyeur is watching a private act without permission.
- *Exhibitionistic disorder:* The erotic interest in exposing one's genitals to others without their explicit consent.
- *Frotteuristic disorder:* The erotic interest in rubbing against someone without their explicit consent.

(All of these disorders have one thing in common: There is no consent from the other person involved.)

- *Sexual masochism disorder:* The erotic interest in being bound, abused, beaten, or having pain or humiliation afflicted.
- *Sexual sadism disorder:* The erotic interest in hurting others.

(Many people enjoy a little pain during sexual encounters, but not to the point of actually being hurt or seriously hurting someone else for enjoyment.)

- *Pedophilic disorder:* The erotic interest in children before puberty.
- *Fetishistic disorder:* The erotic interest in objects such as clothing, footwear, rubber, or leather.
- *Transvestic disorder:* The erotic interest in wearing clothes that are typically linked to the opposite sex.

The bestselling trilogy *Fifty Shades of Grey* not only normalized but celebrated bondage, discipline, dominance, and submission sex play, essentially creating an opportunity for many who had repressed their desires out of fear of being "different." At the same time, the portrayal is also criticized as not representing the actual "rules" involved in kink. Kink sex play is never coercive, and the rules are clearer than portrayed in the multimillion-dollar movies. A 2015 article from *The Atlantic* summarizes the controversy, rightly stating, "there are healthy, ethical ways to consensually combine sex and pain. All of them require self-knowledge, communication skills, and emotional maturity in order to make the sex safe and mutually gratifying. The problem is that *Fifty Shades* casually associates hot sex with violence, but without any of this context."

The rapid rise of the erotic book market may have contributed to a broader acceptance of nontraditional sexual expression. According to Yahoo Finance, erotica sales in 2020 rose 823% in Australia. For the past two decades, US sales of erotica, both self-published and trade titles, have increased year after year, according to an article on the economics of erotica on CNBC. The benefit of this is that it allows people to identify with their sexual interests in a less judgmental or isolated fashion; the downside is if it leads to increased risk taking.

An article in Healthline in 2019 cited research that one in four adults expressed an interest in fetish play and one in three expressed at least a passing interest in voyeurism. Another relatively common phenomenon that can increase someone's risk for infections is participating in "play parties" or orgies. The same article cited 1 in 5 men and 1 in 10 women had participated in group sex.

Orgies have been around since Roman times. In an article in *Psychology Today* in 2019, the author chronicles the long history of "Spring Break" and sexual celebrations to enhance the fertility of coming crops, tracking orgies from Egypt to Greece to Rome to our present-day practices. However, by definition, group sex puts you in a higher-risk category simply by exposing you to multiple partners and their body fluids. "Swinging," also known as "the Lifestyle," refers to open relationships that might involve multiple partners together or separately in time and space. I have personally seen a significant upward trend in older adults having consensual, thoughtful sex outside of their otherwise monogamous marriage. There is even a website for swinging seniors in Florida with information on the over 300 "lifestyle" clubs and vacations available nationwide. Interested? Look for those cute pineapples that adorn mailboxes and front doors—if they are upside down, that's an invitation to swing!

One of my colleagues, Dr. Landi Cranstoun, has developed expertise in the world of kinks, and I asked her to share some of the ways kinks in the older population might create difficulties or opportunities. She shared that one unique thing about kink and aging is that kink activities can be physically demanding, which could result in injury or the need to make modifications due to aging or chronic illness. On the positive side, she shared that kink communities tend to be pretty accepting of a wide range of body types and ages, including older adults. On the negative side, kink-oriented people tend to experience high degrees of discrimination, as well as lots of anticipated stigma in medical situations. Finally, she shared that kink can provide a way to be sexual/erotic for people for whom genital sex is undesirable (perhaps due to the lack of vaginal lubrication or difficulty with erection) since kink doesn't necessarily need to involve genitals.

She shared some specific examples of how aging might complicate this type of sexual activity and create a need for alterations in how to engage in these erotic adventures:

- A couple in their 70s, one of whom was a master of single-tail whipping (I had to look this up—think dog-sled whips), had a long-term partner who was submissive but had had bilateral knee replacements and could no longer kneel. They had to adapt their practice to find a submissive position that would allow his knees to bend.
- A woman in her 60s had been active in kinky sex play in her 20s, but she had not been for decades. She had a new partner who was interested in trying it. Excited to go back to flogging, where she was able to punish her partner with a whip, she was stopped short with the sudden onset of shoulder pain. She had torn her rotator cuff, which required shoulder surgery and months of rehab.
- A man in his 70s had always been a "top" (he was the inserting partner) until he lost erectile function. Despite aggressive attempts to restore function, nothing was successful. Rather than give up on sex, he embraced a new kink identity as a "toppled

top." Shifting his focus away from being the dominant one, he accepted "being punished" as a substitute and would advertise his orifices as available to be used at will. For him, unable to top anymore, he became a bottom (the receptive partner) and embraced feeling dominated, which felt erotic and exciting.

If you are someone who participates in kinks or paraphilic behaviors, or any bread-and-butter contortionist sex for that matter, having awareness of your body's limitations with age is important. Orthopedic issues are very common risks in later-life sex for everyone, and sometimes accommodations must be made.

As you saw in Dr. Cranstoun's last example, one person went from being relatively low risk for sexually transmitted infection (a top) to incredibly high risk (bottom) when he made accommodations for erectile dysfunction. If he was not sharing his sexual risks with his health care provider, they would undoubtedly miss out on critical screening tests and early diagnosis for infection. This not only would have put him at risk but all his partners as well.

One of my urology colleagues shared that the field of urology had seen an increasing incidence of trauma and retained foreign bodies from "urethral play." This is sexual activity that involves placing things (liquids and solids) into the male urethra where, unfortunately, they can then get lodged in the bladder. I like to describe the urethra as a "one-way street." The risk of infection and injury is significant if things go in the wrong direction. A study in the *Journal of Urology* in 2010 found that 24% of male respondents stated they had performed some form of urethral investigation for pleasure.

This urologist shared a story about an older gentleman who came in for lower abdominal pain in the area of his bladder. After failing to be diagnosed by his primary care physician and an urgent care, and the only abnormality on exam was a small amount of blood in his urine, urology had been called to help make the elusive diagnosis. Concerned about kidney stones, they took an X-ray. Instead of stones, they found his bladder was full of bullets. Yes, you read that right: bullets! The small metal projectile of bullets filled his bladder. He would insert them for sexual pleasure, and he hoped eventually they would come out with urination but was too embarrassed to confess the likely cause of his pain. It would have been so much easier if the patient had just said, "I have had pain ever since I have spent the last several years working bullets inside my penis."

My urology colleague went on to share that urethral play can take a very dangerous turn and cause permanent trauma. I asked him what types of things he had encountered being inserted into the penis, and he shared that ballpoint pens and aerosolized tire inflator content were both high on his list of unusual urethral trauma he had witnessed in his career.

## Sex Toys

Every health care provider I know has a good foreign-body story. Some have dozens. There are the countless stories from "old timers" who would be called to the ER to investigate leaves growing out of vaginas. The flora was most often due to baking potatoes being used as pessaries, a common country home remedy, to hold the falling uterus back inside the vagina. Leaving them in too long in that warm, moist environment caused them to sprout. A medical-grade pessary is made out of inert plastic or silicone, but they were not always available a few decades ago. Retained tampon stories are the horror and dread of many adolescents and, having had to go spelunking for a few myself, the sooner you can get them out, the better! There are numerous ways and places people can put inanimate objects inside of themselves. It is the stories of sex toys going missing that I will share now.

One of my colleagues is a vulvar specialist, and she shared a foreign-body story of a late-night consultation in the emergency room.

A sweet couple had come to a local resort in her area to celebrate an impressive anniversary milestone. As a gift for his wife, the man produced a pair of Kegel balls (also known as Ben Wa balls, sex beads, sex eggs). These are used for two main purposes: as a tool to strengthen the muscles of the pelvic floor and for sexual pleasure. In many ways, the first leads to the second as well. By placing these balls in the vagina, the muscles contract. Think of it like sit-ups for the vagina! Strengthening these muscles can assist with urinary incontinence (bladder leaking) and enhance the sensation and intensity of orgasm. Usually made out of silicone or metal, some come with an attachment to help pull them out while others are just weighted balls. (Interested in learning more? Health.com has a nice review article on their picks for the best products.)

Slightly skeptical, but not wanting to disappoint her husband, she proceeded to put the balls in her vagina, and they left for dinner. Like lifting weights, you don't go for a 500-pound set your first day in the gym, and it doesn't take untrained pelvic muscles long to fatigue from holding the balls inside. The added sensation of things rattling around in there can lead one to feeling amorous as it did with this couple. Upon return to her room, he went to retrieve them.

He couldn't get them out.

Panic began to set in as she tried to get them out, and she could not either.

At this point the fatigued muscles started cramping (think shin splints after a hard run but in your vagina). Every time they tried to remove them, her muscles would spasm painfully, which ultimately led to a visit to the local emergency room. Once there, much to her horror, the ER doctor did a pelvic exam but he also could not get them out. The slippery balls and the muscle spasms kept them firmly in place. He called the gynecology resident on call, who was also unsuccessful. Finally, my colleague was called to assist. Success finally came after the patient was "put to sleep" with conscious sedation, which allowed the muscles to finally relax, and the benign little balls were easily retrieved.

Removed and cleaned, my colleague handed them to the husband with a cheerful, "Happy Anniversary!"

She remembers his hang-dog expression as he lamented, "After this, she will never let me have sex with her again."

I had a similar task of retrieving a lost foreign body when I was working in an urgent care. A younger couple came in, slightly intoxicated and giggling, because a sex toy had "broken off" in her vagina, and they could not get it out. In fact, the silicone smooth end was inside her vagina and, like our Ben Wa friends, every time I tried to retrieve the slippery device her muscles would go into spasm. She would start writhing on the table and yelling out in agony. The intensity of the muscle cramps literally gripped my hand as I tried to secure the elusive toy. She also ended up in the ER to receive conscious sedation in order to remove the silicone pleasure.

Stories of foreign bodies in medicine are not uncommon and do not discriminate based on age. Where we get into real trouble can be the rectum. Unlike the vagina, which is a dead-end street for anything bigger than sperm or bacteria, things in the rectum can actually keep moving up and in through a great long highway of intestines. While urethral play can land things in the bladder, the rectum just keeps going. My best advice is to use caution with what you put inside of you, don't leave things in for long, and have a plan for retrieval.

The sex toy market is hopping worldwide, and between 2019 and 2026 it is expected to grow into a $56.7 billion industry, according to Statista. The article goes onto state that in the United States, 65% of adult women own a sex toy, the majority of which are vibrators or rubber penises. Sex toys are used for a variety of reasons, whether for personal gratification or to spice up a bedroom that has gotten dull. One important aspect of sex toys I touched on earlier is the potential transmission of sexually transmitted infections. When toys are shared in real time, with collective warm body fluids from more than one person, it is the perfect means of passing along viruses, fungi, and bacteria. To prevent this, using a barrier method with the toy can help, and careful cleaning between uses is critical. Cleaning with warm water and a gentle soap and then drying completely is a good standard. Using stronger anti-infectives and chemicals can erode the components of the toy or create cracks that can harbor infection (or result in things breaking when you least expect it).

Accidental trauma, orthopedic injuries, retained foreign bodies, and other physical genital misadventures are all ways to land yourself in the ER. Being mindful of making smart choices will decrease your risk of needing medical attention after a roll in the hay. There are plenty of other techniques for practicing sex safely that will save you the embarrassment and cost of sex gone awry.

At the very least, you should know your risk category and get checked as frequently (or infrequently) as recommended based on the prevailing guidelines published by the CDC. Medicare pays for the vast majority of these labs and, if for some reason they don't, go to your local health department STD Clinic. It is your responsibility to keep your house clean so you are not the vector spreading infection to others. Very few people want to be Typhoid Mary. Don't forget that all body parts that have been exposed to another person's genitals and body fluids need to be checked for asymptomatic infection. If you go to your PCP and they shrug you off or are not interested in doing STD testing, consider two things: change health care providers or show them what the CDC recommendations say about screening based on your risk factors.

### Vaccines and Active Disease Prevention Options

In chapters 5 and 6, we talked about HPV and the vaccination that is available to prevent genital warts and cancers. We've already discussed the benefit from PrEP (pre-exposure prophylaxis) to prevent HIV infection, but there are other vaccines that can help keep you protected from infections and STDs.

Most people can benefit from the hepatitis A and B vaccines, if you do not have immunity already, so it's something you should talk to your health care provider about. Anyone who travels internationally should strongly consider the hepatitis A vaccine—while it is not sexually transmitted, hepatitis A is rampant in many countries where eating the food can put you at risk.

There are many vaccines you should have on a schedule. Even though the flu, pneumonia, shingles, and COVID vaccines do not necessarily prevent STDs, you sure won't feel like having sex if you are in the hospital with one of these infections. Don't forget what we learned about subtle and sneaky herpes and HPV infections: A serious illness can trigger a relapse of previously dormant HSV and HPV infections. The healthiest choice is to make sure you are kept up to date on all the vaccines you are eligible for.

## Power in Numbers

We are in the home stretch. You have learned so much! You have undoubtedly had the occasional thought pass through your mind, "*No way!* She is making that up!" or "I seriously doubt that's even possible," or "That is too crazy to actually be true." But I assure you that the stories I have shared are all real people that I, or a trusted colleague, have had the privilege of caring for. In recent years, I have witnessed a concerning pattern coming through the doors of the STD clinic, accompanied by even more concerning statistics. There are consistent increases in STDs in our country, each year outpacing the prior year, despite the fact that many STDs are completely preventable or at the very least, manageable.

Imagine if everyone read this book and digested the content mentally. What if they adhered to the basic advice of thoughtful partner choices, barrier methods, screening tests at appropriate intervals, and going to the doctor and speaking openly and honestly about symptoms, concerns, and risks? There would be no need for the book anymore. All it takes is one "Romeo" to stay ahead of their sexual health to prevent a whole trail of Benvolios from falling. You can be that hero, the one who breaks the cycle and puts an end to a series of infections being spread from one person to the next, by getting a timely diagnosis and alerting partners.

What's holding you back?

## CHAPTER 10

# Ready, Set, Sex

Living a sex revolution, being sex savvy
Is the smartest sex solution

I ASKED ONE of my STD clinic colleagues, I have enjoyed working for nearly two decades, if she had any good STD stories to share for my book about STDs in older adults. She immediately laughed with a snort and said I could share her personal story about "ugly sex."

"Ugly sex? Do I want to hear this?" I asked warily.

We were standing in the clinician workspace with nurses bustling around us, setting up labs for afternoon clinic. She proceeded to jovially tell me about a recent sexual encounter she had with her husband of many years. She was tucked into bed with her hard plastic night guard retainer in place, drool already collecting at the corners of her mouth. The retainer created a gap between her top and bottom teeth, so her words came out in a drunken lisp. She had already said good night and turned off the lights. Her husband, likewise, was settled in and hooked up to his CPAP machine. He was making strangely soothing "Darth Vader" breathing sounds. She began drifting off.

The next thing she knew, he was poking her in the back.

"Hey, hey, you still awake?" He wheezed between bursts of air escaping through the catcher's mask of his CPAP.

She turned her head toward him, without rolling over.

"I am not getting up to take this retainer out," she said definitively through her plastic-congested mouth.

He started fussing with her nightgown and replied with staccato CPAP bursts, "You don't. Have. To say. Anything. Just roll. Over. Honey."

She could only imagine what they must've looked like, him strapped into his CPAP and her drooling with a big retainer in her mouth. She contemplated for a moment but ultimately decided that although their aging sexual life may look unattractive as she approached 60, it was still well worth it.

She happily delayed her bedtime.

Sex doesn't have to look pretty to feel good. The Sexual Revolution of the present day is a terrific thing! Humans are sexual beings by nature, and while some are happy with that part of their lives sun-setting in their older years, there are others who deeply desire to continue it or resume it after a pause. Individuals crave intimacy at different levels, from those who are only looking for a casual hookup to those content with one lifelong mate.

Over the years, I have spoken with many older adults about their sexual desires and urges. One patient who was in her early 70s shared this sentiment: "My partner died four years ago. I have to say I've discovered I'm perfectly happy living by myself. I'm really pretty happy with my own company. There have been times in my life when I was really, really lonely living alone, but I don't feel that way now."

Another woman, also in her 70s, shared, "I had sex too soon after my husband died two years ago. I wasn't ready. It ruined a good friendship. I was so lonely, but that wasn't the answer."

There is no right or wrong level of sexual interest and there is no shame or judgment, no matter where you fall on that spectrum. Sexual prowess may vary with age, hormones, and external circumstances, and sexual appetites can change drastically from partner to partner. Some people are innately more sexual beings than others and enjoy great health late in life. Others have suffered through and survived cancer treatments that have left their bodies and their hormone levels permanently altered. Chronic disease leaves others with their sexual function permanently impaired, but that does not mean closing the door on intimacy. There are plenty of other ways to be intimate. There is a wonderful book by Emily Nogoski, a sex therapist, that I learned about from my vulvar specialist colleague. She recommends all older women read Nogoski's *Come As You Are*, which delves into sexuality and important body issues for women. If you are a woman who is struggling with late-life intimacy, you might consider picking it up.

## What Has Not Been Covered

There are far more rare STDs, but thus far I have focused on the things you are most likely to encounter in the United States. There are some countries that boast a menu of sexually transmitted options that is more expansive. Having unprotected sex with a sex worker in certain countries, for example, is a pretty bad idea. We did not cover chancroid or lymphogranulum venereum (LGV) in any detail in this book because the incidence is exceptionally low in the United States. They are rare enough that the 2021 STI Guidelines almost left them out altogether. They are bacterial infections caused by the bacteria *H. ducreyi* and *C. trachomatis* (a particular strain of chlamydia), respectively. Chancroid falls into the category of a genital ulcer disease and was only reported in three people in the entire country in 2018 (fig. 10.1).

LGV is also rarely reported, but the incidence is hard to measure since the cause is a particularly virulent strain of chlamydia that sets up a chronic infection in the lymphatic system. It can cause swollen lymph nodes that burst and the destruction of the genital mucosa, leaving severe scarring. In 2016, there was an outbreak in Michigan and all 38 infections were in HIV-positive men. Interestingly, LGV is beginning to be implicated in cases of proctitis in both older adults and those infected with HIV, so it may be an infection to watch for in the future.

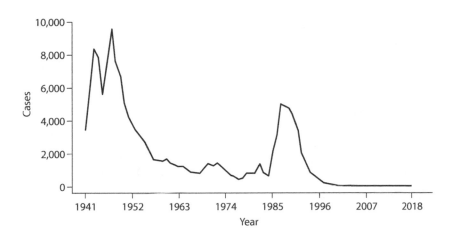

FIGURE 10.1.
Reported cases of chancroid by year in the United States from 1941 to 2018.
*Source:* cdc.gov

"Out On a Limb"
I'm going to go out on a limb
And say the odds of safe sex are grim.
The news says, Eureka!
That rascally Zika,
Spreads by sex him-to-her, her-to-him.

There has also been an increase in the number of tropical viral illnesses and other infections that can be sexually transmitted. Zika, as you have undoubtedly read about in the news, is a tropical mosquito-borne illness that causes a tragic birth defect in countless babies around the world, most notably in Brazil. It has been demonstrated that transmission from person-to-person creates a concern, particularly in pregnant women. The virus can spread from the mother to the unborn fetus, and from male to female through unprotected sex. Today's guidelines continue that if a male travels to an area with Zika, the recommendation from the CDC is they use condoms for three months upon return to prevent transmitting to a woman who might become pregnant.

Ebola, one of the deadliest viral infections, has strangled parts of Africa in the past several years. It is transmitted from an infected person to another through bodily fluids. Studies have shown that it continues to live in the testicular fluid of men for months after someone is infected and actually survives. Interestingly, while it can be transmitted by a man in semen, it does not appear to be transmittable from a woman's vaginal fluids. Suffice it to say, these occurrences are rare and are not the infections that keep the average STD health care provider awake at night.

## Sex in a Pandemic

When I started writing this book, I could not have imagined that I would be adding a section on having sex during a pandemic. But coronavirus (COVID-19) quickly began to spread around the globe, and virtually overnight our world changed. I have had the privilege to work for the Department of Health & Human Services in North Carolina through the pandemic and have led efforts to rapidly develop and deploy telehealth, increase testing sites when they were hard to acquire, and operationalize the rapid distribution of vaccine across the state equitably. It certainly created a diversion from thinking about STDs!

The good news is, COVID-19 is not sexually transmitted—well, from the body fluid exchange standpoint—but it sure is contagious. With pandemic protocols in place for many months, including masking recommendations when within 6 feet of one another, dating and intimacy became an enormous challenge. So COVID-19 was, in an indirect way, sexually transmitted. If you were having sex with a new partner during a pandemic of this magnitude, you were running the extremely high risk of exposing yourself to the virus or spreading asymptomatic infection. I have often wondered if there are people out there wearing N95 masks while having sex. If so, we are taking protection to a whole new level! As if all the STDs in the world weren't enough to contend with!

Many people did not let the pandemic slow them down. Some continued to use dating apps and instead of face-to-face meetings, arrange for virtual dates. Others met partners outdoors only where the risk of transmission was less. Still others didn't buy into the pandemic hype and continued as if nothing was different. Being cooped up at home meant some couples rekindled their sex lives while others found the stress and constant togetherness squelched any flames of passion. The pandemic saw drug and alcohol use increase, and unintentional overdose deaths from opioids rise, so it's fair to assume those struggling with sex addiction continued to engage in high-risk encounters as well. I took care of a taxi driver once who informed me that had sex several times a day, every day, and often with different people. If someone could not afford the fare, he accepted sex of all kinds in payment. I wondered how he handled the restrictions and limitations that COVID-19 presented.

It seems that quarantine life didn't stop people from having sexual relations and spreading STDs. Surprisingly, patient demand in the STD clinic that I work at did not decrease during the pandemic. Just recently, a handful of my patients who were over 50 all received a diagnosis of a sexually transmitted infection (not a single "worried penis" in the lot). Genital warts, trichomonas, and herpes led the charge in these patients, as they often do in the older demographic. In fact, everyone I saw that day tested positive for an STD. This tells me that sexual activity, as a whole, has not taken a back seat despite a global health crisis. And if these patients aren't protecting themselves by wearing condoms, I'm quite certain they are not protecting themselves by wearing masks. In fact, I think it would be safe to say I have diagnosed more new cases of HIV in 2022 than I did all together in the past decade.

One unintended consequence of the national response to the pandemic was shortages in all facets of medical treatment, including in the STD world, which potentially set the stage for a concerning surge in post-pandemic STD rates. Health departments across the country were forced to shift their staff to focus on COVID-19 testing, contact tracing, and COVID-19 vaccinations, leaving other clinics abandoned. Labs around the country had similar split priorities. The machines normally used for STD testing were re-prioritized for COVID-19 instead. The national shortages of the reagent to process the NAAT tests for chlamydia, gonorrhea, and trichomonas were seen widely. Lab staff were diverted to COVID-19 activities. The result was multifold: limited access to clinics because staff were diverted, fewer tests being done for both screening and diagnostic purposes around the country, and diminished resources for follow-up. Those harboring asymptomatic infections across the country will result in a veritable tsunami of STDs, equipped with a copious number of complications, as lab capacity returns to normal and people re-engage in care.

## Where There Is Rhyme, There Is Rap

I am a physician, but I am also a rapper. I am not necessarily a very good rapper, but I love rap. My first rap lyrics came sometime in late middle school. Not long after when I was in college, my best friend since middle school, Susan, and I became the "Two Mid-evil Crew," serfs rapping Shakespeare and introducing the scenes in the elementary schools as part of a college literature class. The innumerable thank-you letters from the young children consistently proved that The Rapping Serfs were the headliner and highlight of their day. I went on to rap in medical school and residency about any number of topics: hyperkalemia, leukemia, post-trauma Foley catheters—everything is better with rhyme. I have never stopped rapping or rhyming. I remember being frustrated on my OB rotations in residency by all the women who were insistent on vaginal deliveries. There was a huge cultural shift in the early 2000s when women would risk the health of their babies in order to deliver "naturally" (vaginally), rather than with a repeat C-section. As a result, I formulated the rap "Desperate Vaginas" on a punchy, sleep-deprived, call night. Rap and rhyme are part of my DNA, which I blame wholesale on the influence of Shel Silverstein and all the old-school rap artists who molded me.

I embarked on my first STD rap video in 2015, titled "Off to the STD Clinic You Go," based off of an old-school hip-hop song called "Principal's Office" by Young MC, which had topped the charts in 1989. I was giving lectures at public speaking events for youth groups, schools, and colleges about STDs and was amazed at the lack of education these kids brought to the table. They were old enough to know that they had definitely been learning this material in school, but it was clear that they were not absorbing it. Were my words going in one ear and out the other? If so, how could I reach them differently, I pondered.

Rap seemed like a great answer.

I wrote the rap and recorded it in the basement of a West Asheville house with help from my colleague, Dr. Rob Fields, and a friend of his who enjoyed playing music, Dr. Andy Runkle. I shot the video with the help of my (then) preteen and teen sons who dragged a spider-web-laden shop light out of the garage and helped me set up the filming across town. For locations, we used my clinic, a neighbor's office, and my neighbor's house. In one scene, after I "make it rain" condoms, all the kids would scramble around on the floor collecting them for the next cut. Making it rain condoms is no easy task! Like many parental lookbacks, it now occurs to me that perhaps that was inappropriate.

The local news picked up my first rap video and featured a piece on it, thanks to reporter Frank Kracher, who never looked away just because a topic was edgy. The video was popular and several school districts wanted to use it, but it would not pass their "Internet filters" because of the content involving s-e-x. It died on the vine, but it serves as a great icebreaker to use at the beginning of STD talks. It's still out there on YouTube if you'd like to see it (fig. 10.2). After shooting this video, I received some feedback expressing concern that I had engaged in cultural appropriation because I was wearing a wig. I took that feedback and have never worn that wig again.

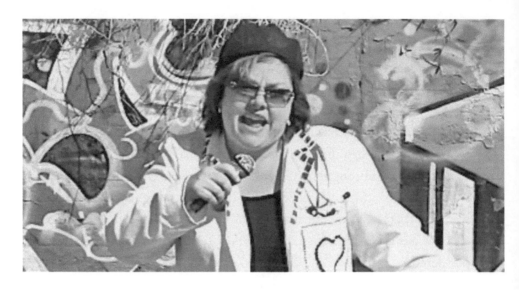

FIGURE 10.2.
A still from the "STDs Never Get Old" video, March 2017.
*Source:* Author; https://www.youtube.com/watch?v=wMFRM1bkEDg

It was around 2014 when I began to observe the trend of increased STDs in the older population. My clinics experienced a subtle shift from the extraordinarily rare adult over 50 to every clinic having several adults over 50 and some even into their early 80s. This coincided with what the media was reporting regarding some prominent retirement communities like The Villages, in Florida. These senior communities were also seeing a staggering spike in STD rates.

The AARP covered this phenomenon: "In Central Florida, where The Villages and other retirement communities sprawl across several counties, reported cases of syphilis and chlamydia increased 71% among those fifty-five and older." The data were showing up in the media everywhere, from *Forbes*, to AARP, to USNews.com, remarking on the increase in STDs in the older population.

I found these stats to be very interesting. It validated that the trend I was observing was widespread. I decided to do more digging. According to an article written by *U.S. News* in 2018, "A recent analysis of patients on athenahealth's network found that patients over age 60 account for the biggest increase of in-office treatments for sexually transmitted infections."

While preparing for a presentation that I periodically gave to about 800 family doctors on STDs, I decided to crunch the data for STDs in the older population in North Carolina. We were seeing a year-over-year increase in the most common STDs for five years running. The numbers were not huge, but they were consistently rising. I was not losing my mind. What does one do when they have something important to say and are seeing such an alarming trend? Obviously, you write a rap song and record a rap video!

This time I took the 1990's hit "Ice, Ice Baby" by Vanilla Ice to the next level, but I changed it to "Safe Sex, Baby." To be clear, I never said I was a good singer or rapper, but my son Eli, a middle schooler at the time, sang in several choruses and had a beautiful voice, so he offered to do the refrain for my recording. Once again, I recruited family and friends to be my "talent" for this home production.

I wrote this rap over the course of a long road trip to Washington, DC. My friend Susan (remember Susan, my Shakespeare rapper friend?) accompanied me, and we spent the drive plotting out how to shoot the different scenes. Her career has been on the directing side of TV and movies, and her longtime boyfriend, Will, was a professional camera operator. A few weeks after our DC drive, we shot the entire video in one weekend. At the time, I was an executive in a health system, and they would not give me permission to shoot the video on their property. I went back to my residency program, MAHEC, which cared for retirement communities and had a strong geriatrics focus. They were more than happy to share their offices for filming on a weekend. One of my colleagues from residency owned a local pharmacy, and he gave me permission to film "the condom scene" (by far the best scene of the video) at his pharmacy. My mom and I recruited friends, neighbors, and family members. We had a whirlwind weekend of shooting!

The following week, I spent long hours editing the video and sound to get the final product polished and perfected. The title of the video came from a Facebook post where my soon-to-be brother-in-law proposed "STDs Never Get Old."

It was a (w)rap!

I reached out to my friend and local news station reporter at WLOS, Frank Kracher, and asked him if he would be interested in shooting a local story about STDs in the older population. Frank has superb storytelling skills, and I trusted him to help raise awareness for the video. When my video aired on the local news, it generated so much buzz! Everyone was talking about it. "STDs Never Get Old" got picked up by the network! The next thing I knew, my mom's friends were emailing her to say they had seen her and dad on something about STDs on the local news around the country. This was completely unexpected. The video was featured on a game show on Comedy Central, where my poor father's face was frozen on a huge screen looking gleeful after being slipped a condom by a "younger" woman. My entertaining, but educational message was circulating, not just around the country, but around the world, at lightning speed. The video had gone viral.

On a Thursday, I was invited to fly out to London to be a guest on *The Last Laugh* the next night (turns out I would have been on with Michael Bolton), but I had clinic the next day and two teen boys and was not able to drop everything and hop on a plane across the ocean. I had to decline the invitation. I was interviewed with iHeartRadio and SiriusXM radio and had the story of my video written about in magazines, newspapers, and websites around the globe. A viral video company reached out to me and wanted to buy the rights to the video, but I declined, to their great distress. They can be quite persistent! I explained the purpose of the video was public education, not profit. I did not want to sign away the rights for profit. I was willing to share the video with any media organization that wanted to cover the video, at no charge. If I am totally honest, I was also a little terrified Vanilla Ice would sue me for taking his pop hit and bastardizing it by rhyming about infected genitals, but I am happy to say I never heard from him.

I have countless lyrics written for more rap videos to come, but time is a fickle thing and my day job takes well more than 40 hours a week. During the pandemic, it was closer to 60 to 80 hours a week. My twist on "It's Tricky," by Run DMC, has not been recorded yet, but it will be a good one when I can find a minute. Keep an ear out for it!

I never expected to be a household name or a viral sensation, but I have welcomed the slew of opportunities that have come from my videos' success. I have even been identified in public a couple times as "that rapping STD doctor," much to my children's horror. The attention enables me to broaden my audience and expand my message. More importantly, even though people are getting a good laugh out of the video, I know they are also learning from it. Plus, it makes a great icebreaker as I warm up an audience for a public speaking event. I can take pride in knowing that I am helping bring attention to the need for sex safe at all ages. Even if only one person watches the videos and heeds my cautions, it is absolutely worth it. The videos led me here, to being given the chance to educate all of you reading this book. And if you're still with me here—thanks for staying with me to the end! You are now practically an expert on the subject of STDs and safe sex!

## Pulling It All Together

Rather than feel anxious after our time together, I hope you feel empowered and armed with knowledge. Whether you are happily abstinent or actively sexual or find yourself somewhere in the middle of that continuum, I hope this book has supplied you with the best methods for avoiding, recognizing, or managing sexually transmitted infections and achieving overall sexual health. You can now serve as a resource for others who might be swimming in these shark-infested sexual waters.

The US Centers for Disease Control and Prevention says that the rapid increase in people contracting STDs must be confronted. Getting the data out into the world is the first step. I have spent over 20 years diagnosing and treating sexually transmitted infections, and I will tell you that I have never—truly, never—seen someone happy to receive an STD diagnosis. It is more than the physical discomfort that sexually transmitted infections can cause; the emotional toil can be significant. It can be stressful. It can feel shameful. It is always disruptive. The good news is the vast majority of infections are completely and totally avoidable with conscientious attention to risks and safety. The first step is understanding the lay of the land, which you are now well acquainted with.

Go forth and be active! Embrace the Golden Years, and recapture or unleash that youthful essence and frolic in intimacy! There is no shame in your ongoing sexuality; there is only shame in failing to care for yourself and others.

"Many Thanks"
You made it through this creation!
My STD heart is filled with elation.
My story's all told—
I hope you are sold—
So sexual health is yours for the duration.

# Acknowledgments

This book has been brewing in my mind for several years, and I have a lot of people to thank for getting it out of my head and onto paper. A heartfelt thanks goes specifically to the following people:

- Marilyn Thiet, an amazing professional coach gifted to me through the leadership of Dr. Jill Hoggard Green, as part of a leadership program developed for executives at Mission Health System; Marilyn helped me find the voice and clarity to discern my next steps.
- My Rap Video Crew: Susan Walter, my BFF since way back, for her directing prowess and the hours of brainstorming on the long drive home from the first Women's March in Washington, DC; Will Hand, our cameraman; and all the amazing family and friends who were the talent—especially for my dad, James Brown, a quiet and private man, who only months before dying had his face plastered on Comedy Central gleefully accepting a condom from a faux paramour.
- The people who make the difference along the way, like Frank Kracher, the WLOS reporter who helped launch my "STDs Never Get Old" video; Dr. Chris DeRienzo, my first boss, who was simultaneously younger and smarter than me, and to add insult to injury, got his first book done before me, dang it.
- My sweet boys, Jacob and Eli, "extras" on raps and videos and "victims" of my STD talks in every school (and family meal) they've attended since puberty.
- To the many men and women whose voices contributed to this book—you know who you are, and I thank you for your willingness to speak your truth. For my colleagues who contributed stories of their own, gave advice, and took this around the final corner: Dr. Maureen Murphy, Dr. Christie Posner, Dr. Rhett Brown, Dr. Kiran Sigmon, Dr. Suzanne Dixon, Dr. Matt Young, Dr. Tom Belt, Dr. Jessica Triche, Dr. Victoria Mobely, and Dr. Emily Diznoff.

- To my lay editors, researchers, and "connectors": my mom, Linda Brown; my mother-in-law, Jennifer Dowler; Aunt Sarah; Uncle Jed; and all the others.
- To my sister, and Irish twin, Dr. Mitchell Brown, who has written countless books before me and talked me off the ledge when I "lost" my drafts in the depths of my computer.
- To the village it takes to keep me afloat not already mentioned: my BFFs Jackie and Marc, Ruth and David, Dennis and Gina, and most of all, my incredibly patient husband and high school sweetheart, Jared.
- Finally, to my agents, editors, and enthusiastic coaches, Kelly Thomas and Regina Brooks from Serendipity Literary Agency, who were willing to take a chance on an edgy topic and a middle-aged, overweight, white rapper.

# Appendix

### "STDs Never Get Old"

Yo, It's RapDoctorD, Let's Kick It!

Safe Sex, Baby
Safe Sex, Baby
Safe Sex, Baby
Safe Sex, Baby

All right, stop! Collaborate and listen
Rap Dr. D's rap intention
Callin' out all ya fellas and la-dies
Cause STDs are tearin' through folks in their 80s.
Can you really help bein' sex kittens?
Why can't you wear your little love mittens?
Gotta be safe, cause sex has gotten risky.
No shame bein' a freak, and gettin' a little frisky.
DANG! Yo body's a temple
Keepin' safe not always so simple.
Sex indiscretions lead to depression
No matter how you like it condoms give the best
protection.
Love it, or leave it, hormones start to flag.
Things dry up and your tail can lose that wag.
If that is a problem, lube may solve it
See your family doc if it doesn't resolve it.

Safe Sex, Baby
Safe Sex, Baby

Safe Sex, Baby
Safe Sex, Baby

Vaginal atrophy is something.
A sex catastrophe it can be the real thing.
Quick to the point, to the point I'm making.
Lubrication's key and you know I'm not faking.
Trauma, from guys' erections,
Tears thin skin without protection.
Listen up and learn from this lection
If you don't want a nasty groin infection.

Aging! It's just a normal stage.
We all gotta get on the same safe sex page.
Fellas on standby wantin' more than say hi
Should you stop? Or should you just drive by?
Wait till they're checked at an STD shop
Check things out from the bottom to the top!
Your sex life can be later and stronger.
Thanks, Viagra, boy parts work longer.
Livin' a sex revolution
Being sex savvy is the smartest sex solution.
So let's break it down, cougars all around.
All these STDs all the time bein' found.
Bodies! We're just a cafeteria
A cesspool of germs, virus and bacteria.
Once called the clap, gonorrhea's got a rap.
Sleeping around? Probably a trap.
Subtle and sneaky is chlamydia
You may not even know when that bug has gotten into ya.
Syphilis makes a painless little sore
Then you spread it round every time you score.
All are on the scene, back in action,
Tear things up, put your parts in traction.
STDs are a problem, one way to solve it.
See your family doc, maybe they can resolve it.

Safe Sex, Baby
Safe Sex, Baby

Safe Sex, Baby
Safe Sex, Baby

Take heed! I'm an STD poet
I'm Rap Dr. D and I want you to know it.
My town! I see these infections
Give bad news when they are detected.
Sex can be a germ spill.
People aren't safe, for real.
Virus and bacteria, sexually transmitted.
How to be safe? Make sure the condom's fitted.
I'm Rap Dr. D and I wanna help you be
Free of herpes, AIDS, and HPV.
All these STDs really are stealthy
Without 'em your sex life can be healthy.
No lame excuses you know to take precautions.
Rap Dr. Out, hope your golden years are awesome.
If you have a problem and condoms can't solve it
See your family doc; maybe they can resolve it.

# References

**INTRODUCTION.**
**You May Be Wondering Why I Have Called You Here Today**
Fontaine, Mia. "America Has an Incest Problem." *The Atlantic*, January 24, 2013. https://www.theatlantic.com/national/archive/2013/01/america-has-an-incest-problem/272459/.

**CHAPTER 1.**
**Sex in the Twenty-First Century**
Pereto, Alison. "Patients Over 60? Screen for STIs." Athena Health, May 16, 2018. https://www.athenahealth.com/knowledge-hub/clinical-trends/over-60-stis-may-not-be-done-you.

"Sexually Transmitted Infections (STIs)." World Health Organization, November 22, 2021. https://www.who.int/news-room/fact-sheets/detail/sexually-transmitted-infections-(stis).

"At More Than 2 Million, CDC Reports Record High Rates of STDs in U.S." (September 27, 2017). *Infectious Disease Special Edition.* https://www.idse.net/Article/PrintArticle?ArticleId=44706.

"New CDC Report: STDs Continue to Rise in the U.S." Centers for Disease Control and Prevention (CDC), October 8, 2019. https://www.cdc.gov/nchhstp/newsroom/2019/2018-STD-surveillance-report-press-release.html#:~:text=Data%20suggest%20that%20multiple%20factors,and%20gay%20and%20bisexual%20men.

"STDs at Record High, Indicating Urgent Need for Prevention." Centers for Disease Control and Prevention (CDC), September 26, 2017. https://www.cdc.gov/media/releases/2017/p0926-std-prevention.html.

"Sexually Transmitted Infections Treatment Guidelines, 2021." Centers for Disease Control and Prevention (CDC), last updated July 22, 2021, https://www.cdc.gov/std/treatment-guidelines/toc.htm.

Borland, Sophie. "Rising Divorce Rates, Casual Sex and Condoms 'Only Being for the Young' Means STDs Have Soared by 38% in Baby Boomer in 3 Years." *Daily Mail UK*, December 8, 2016.

"CDC Now Recommends All Baby Boomers Receive One-Time Hepatitis C Test." Centers for Disease Control and Prevention (CDC). August 16, 2012.

"HIV and Older Americans." Centers for Disease Control and Prevention (CDC). Last updated January 12, 2022.

"National Overview: Sexually Transmitted Disease Surveillance, 2019." Centers for Disease Control and Prevention (CDC). Last modified April 13, 2021.

Griffiths, Meredith. "Baby Boomers Re-entering Dating Game More Vulnerable to Sexually Transmitted Infections." *ABC News Australia*, January 17, 2018.

Gann, Carrie. "Sex Life of Older Adults and Rising STDs." *ABC News*, February 3, 2012.

Underdown, Simon J., Krishna Kumar, and Charlotte Houldcroft, "Network Analysis of the Hominin Origin of Herpes Simplex Virus 2 from Fossil Data." *Virus Evolution* 3, no. 2 (July 2017). https://doi.org/10.1093/ve/vex026.

Rogers, Kara. *Encyclopedia Britannica*, Sexually Transmitted Disease, Pathology, last modified February 20, 2020. https://www.britannica.com/science/sexually-transmitted-disease.

Comas, Martin E. "Oldest County in U.S.? Sumter County, Thanks to The Villages, a 'Retirement Disney World.'" *Orlando Sentinel*, June 28, 2019.

"QuickFacts: The Villages CDP, Florida." (2021). United States Census Bureau. https://www.census.gov/quickfacts/thevillagescdpflorida.

Jameson, Marni, "Seniors' Sex Lives Are Up—and So Are STD Cases Around the Country." AARP, May 17, 2011. https://www.aarp.org/health/conditions-treatments/news-05-2011/seniors_sex_lives_are_up_and_so_are_std_cases.html.

**CHAPTER 2.**
**The Biology of Aging and Sexually Transmitted Diseases**
Meites, Elissa, Peter G. Szilagyi, Harrell W. Chesson, Elizabeth R. Unger, José R. Romero, and Lauri E. Markowitz. "Human Papillomavirus Vaccination for Adults: Updated Recommendations of the Advisory Committee on Immunization Practices." *Morbidity and Mortality Weekly Report*, Centers for Disease Control and Prevention, August 16, 2019.

Jameson, Marni. "Seniors' Sex Lives Are Up—and So Are STD Cases Around the Country." AARP, May 17, 2011.

Sefton, A. M. "The Great Pox That Was . . . Syphilis." *Journal of Applied Microbiology* 91, no. 4 (October 2001): 592–596, https://doi.org/10.1046/j.1365-2672 .2001.01494.x.

Gelpi, Adriane, and Joseph D. Tucker. "After Venus, Mercury: Syphilis Treatment in the UK before Salvarsan." *Sexually Transmitted Infections* (BMI Journals) 91, no. 1 (January 2015).

"The U.S. Public Health Service Syphilis Study at Tuskegee," Centers for Disease Control and Prevention. Last modified April 22, 2021. https:// www.cdc.gov/tuskegee/timeline.htm.


**CHAPTER 3.**
**The Good, the Bad, and the Ugly**
eHarmony Editorial Team. "10 Online Dating Statistics You Should Know." eHarmony. Last modified March 18, 2021. https://www.eharmony.com /online-dating-statistics/.

Bayly, Lucy. "Golden Oldies: One in 10 Americans Dating Online Is a Baby Boomer." *NBC News*, February 11, 2016.

Stodart, Leah, and Miller Kern, "Best Senior Dating Sites: Dating Over 60 Can Actually Be Fun." *Mashable*, December 21, 2021. https://mashable.com /roundup/best-dating-sites-for-seniors/.

Neely, Leigh, James Combs, Theresa Campbell, and Debbi Kiddy. "The Untold Stories of The Villages." *Lake & Sumter Style*, October 1, 2016. https://www.lakeandsumterstyle.com/the-untold-stories-of-the -villages/.

Vanman, Eric. "We Asked Catfish Why They Trick People Online—It's Not about Money." Phsy.org. Last modified July 26, 2018. https://phys.org /news/2018-07-catfish-people-onlineit-money.html.

Birger, Jon. "Why Dating Apps Are No Way to Find True Love." *Newsweek*, February 2, 2021. https://www.newsweek.com/why-dating-apps-are-no -way-find-true-love-1565682.

Coduto, Kathryn D., Roselyn J. Lee-Won, and Young Min Baek. "Swiping for Trouble: Problematic Dating Application Use among Psychosocially Distraught Individuals and the Paths to Negative Outcomes." *The Journal of Social and Personal Relationships* 37, no. 1 (January 1, 2020): 212–232. https://doi.org/10.1177%2F0265407519861153.

"Sexually Transmitted Infections Prevalence, Incidence, and Cost Estimates in the United States." Centers for Disease Control and Prevention (CDC), last modified, January 25, 2021. https://www.cdc.gov/std/statistics/prevalence -2020-at-a-glance.htm.

Flynn, Hillary, Keith Cousins, and Elizabeth Naismith Picciani. "Tinder Lets Known Sex Offenders Use the App: It's Not the Only One." *ProPublica* and Columbia Journalism Investigations, December 2, 2019. https://www .propublica.org/article/tinder-lets-known-sex-offenders-use-the-app-its -not-the-only-one.

"Chlamydia Screening in Women (CHL)." National Committee for Quality Assurance (NCQA). https://www.ncqa.org/hedis/measures/chlamydia -screening-in-women/.

"Sexually Transmitted Infections Treatment Guidelines, 2021." Centers for Disease Control and Prevention (CDC). Last updated July 22, 2021. https://www.cdc.gov/std/treatment-guidelines/default.htm.

"Ocular Syphilis—Eight Jurisdictions, United States, 2014–2015." *Morbidity and Mortality Weekly Report*, Centers for Disease Control and Prevention. Last modified November 4, 2016. https://www.cdc.gov/mmwr/volumes/65/wr /mm6543a2.htm.

Liu, Hui, Shannon Shen, and Ning Hsieh. "A National Dyadic Study of Oral Sex, Relationship Quality, and Well-Being among Older Couples." *The Journals of Gerontology Series B: Psychological Sciences and Social Sciences* 74, no. 2 (February 2019; published online August 4, 2018): 298–308. https:// doi.org/10.1093/geronb/gby089.

"Virginity Pledges Do Not Work, Yet Another Study Confirms." Guttmacher Institute. Last modified December 30, 2008. https://www.guttmacher.org /article/2008/12/virginity-pledges-do-not-work-yet-another-study -confirms.

## CHAPTER 4.
### Treatable, Curable STDs

Taylor, Ashley. "Cavorting Wee Beasties." *Yale Medicine*, Winter 2014. https:// medicine.yale.edu/news/yale-medicine-magazine/article/cavorting-wee -beasties/.

Owusu-Edusei, Kwame Jr., Harrell W. Chesson, Thomas L. Gift, Guoya Tao, Reena Mahajan, Marie Cherly Banez Ocfemia, and Charlotte K. Kent. (2013, March). The Estimated Direct Medical Cost of Selected Sexually Transmitted Infections in the United States, 2008. *Sexually Transmitted Diseases*, 40(3): 197–201. https://doi.org/1097/OLQ.0b013e318285c6d2.

"Trichomoniasis: Is it always sexually transmitted?" *National Center for Biotechnology Information* 35, no. 2; July–December 2014 PMC4553853, https://doi .org/10.4103/2589-0557.142422, https://www.ncbi.nlm.nih.gov/pmc /articles/PMC4553853/.

"Primary and Secondary Syphilis—United States, 2000–2001." *Morbidity and Mortality Weekly Report*, Centers for Disease Control and Prevention, November 1, 2002 / 51(43): 971–973. https://www.cdc.gov/mmwr/preview /mmwrhtml/mm5143a4.htm.

"Reported STDs in the United States, 2019." CDC Fact Sheet: Reported STDs in the United States, 2019. https://www.cdc.gov/nchhstp/newsroom/docs /factsheets/std-trends-508.pdf.

"Sexually Transmitted Infections Treatment Guidelines, 2021." Centers for Disease Control and Prevention (CDC). Last updated July 22, 2021. https://www.cdc.gov/std/treatment-guidelines/toc.htm.

## CHAPTER 5.
### Treatable, Not Curable STDs

"HPV and Men: Fact Sheet." Centers for Disease Control and Prevention. Last modified January 3, 2022. https://www.cdc.gov/std/hpv/stdfact-hpv-and -men.htm.

"Massive Proportion of World's Population Are Living with Herpes Infection." World Health Organization. Last modified May 1, 2020. https://www.who .int/news/item/01-05-2020-massive-proportion-world-population-living -with-herpes-infection.

"Human Papillomavirus (HPV) Statistics." Centers for Disease Control and Prevention. Last modified April 5, 2021. https://www.cdc.gov/std/hpv /stats.htm.

"Understanding HPV Coverage." Centers for Disease Control and Prevention. Last modified August 23, 2018. https://www.cdc.gov/hpv/partners /outreach-hcp/hpv-coverage.html.

Saslow, Debbie, Kimberly S. Andrews, Deana Manassaram-Baptiste, Robert A. Smith, and Elizabeth T. H. Fontham. "Human Papillomavirus Vaccination 2020 Guideline Update: American Cancer Society Guideline Adaptation." *CA: A Cancer Journal for Clinicians* 70, no. 4 (July/August 2020): 274–280. https://doi.org/10.3322/caac.21616.

"Herpes Simplex Virus." World Health Organization. Last modified May 1, 2020. https://www.who.int/news-room/fact-sheets/detail/herpes-simplex-virus.

"Long-Term Outcome of Severe Herpes Simplex Encephalitis: A Population-Based Observational Study." National Center for Biotechnology Information, September 21, 2015. https://www.ncbi.nlm.nih.gov/pmc/articles /PMC4576407/#CR1.

"Sexually Transmitted Infections Treatment Guidelines, 2021." Centers for Disease Control and Prevention (CDC). https://www.cdc.gov/std /treatment-guidelines/toc.htm.

**CHAPTER 6.**
**Treatable, Incurable, Potentially Life-Limiting STDs**

"CDC Now Recommends All Baby Boomers Receive One-Time Hepatitis C Test." *Morbidity and Mortality Weekly Report*, Centers for Disease Control and Prevention, August 16, 2012. https://www.cdc.gov/nchhstp/newsroom /2012/hcv-testing-recs-pressrelease.html#:~:text=More%20than%20 2%20million%20U.S.,adults%20living%20with%20the%20virus.

"HIV and Older Americans." Centers for Disease Control and Prevention, January 12, 2022. https://www.cdc.gov/hiv/group/age/olderamericans /index.html.

"Diagnoses of HIV Infection Among Adults Aged 50 Years and Older in the United States and Dependent Areas, 2011–2016." Centers for Disease Control and Prevention, *HIV Surveillance Report, Supplemental Report* 23, no. 5. https://www.cdc.gov/hiv/pdf/library/reports/surveillance/cdc-hiv-surveillance-supplemental-report-vol-23-5.pdf.

Saag, Michael S. "CDC: More Americans Die of HCV Than Any Other Infectious Disease." *Infectious Disease News*, June 15, 2016. https://www.healio.com/news/infectious-disease/20160615/cdc-more-americans-die-of-hcv-than-any-other-infectious-disease.

"For Older Adults, Newer Hepatitis C Treatments Are Safe and Effective." Health in Aging. *Journal of the American Geriatrics Society*, Research Summary. November 8, 2019. https://www.healthinaging.org/blog/for-older-adults-newer-hepatitis-c-treatments-are-safe-and-effective/.

"Viral Hepatitis in the United States: Data and Trends." HHS.gov. US Department of Health & Human Services. Office of Infectious Disease and HIV/AIDS Policy (OIDP). June 7, 2016. https://www.hhs.gov/hepatitis/learn-about-viral-hepatitis/data-and-trends/index.html.

"What Is Hepatitis B?" Hepatitis B Foundation. https://www.hepb.org/what-is-hepatitis-b/what-is-hepb/.

"Of Warts, Nuns and Jackalopes: A Brief History of the HPV Vaccine." UNC Healthy Heels. May 24, 2012. https://healthyheels.org/2012/05/24/of-warts-nuns-and-jackalopes-a-brief-history-of-the-hpv-vaccine-draft/.

"HPV-Associated Cancer Diagnosis by Age." Centers for Disease Control and Prevention, December 13, 2021. https://www.cdc.gov/cancer/hpv/statistics/age.htm.

## CHAPTER 7.
### The Great Mimickers: Things That Are Probably *Not* STDs

"Psoriasis Statistics." National Psoriasis Foundation. Last modified October 8, 2020. https://www.psoriasis.org/psoriasis-statistics/.

Meeuwis, Kim A. P., Alison Potts Bleakman, Peter C. M. van de Kerkhof, Yves Dutronc, Carsten Henneges, Lori J. Kornberg, and Alan Menter. "Prevalence of Genital Psoriasis in Patients with Psoriasis." *Journal of Dermatological Treatment* 29, no 8 (December 29, 2018): 754–760. https://pubmed.ncbi.nlm.nih.gov/29565190/.

Kirtschig, Gudula. "Lichen Sclerosus—Presentation, Diagnosis and Management." US National Library of Medicine. National Institutes of Health. *Deutsches Arzteblatt International* 113, no. 19 (May 2016): 337–343. https://www.ncbi.nlm.nih.gov/pmc/articles/PMC4904529/.

Love, Lauren W., Talel Badri, and Michael L. Ramsey. "Pearly Penile Papule." National Center for Biotechnology Information. September 28, 2021. https://www.ncbi.nlm.nih.gov/books/NBK442028/.

## CHAPTER 8.
### Staying on Top of Things (So to Speak)

"The National Health Expenditure Accounts—Historical." CMS.gov, Centers for Medicare & Medicaid Services. Last modified December 15, 2021. https://www.cms.gov/Research-Statistics-Data-and-Systems/Statistics-Trends-and-Reports/NationalHealthExpendData/NationalHealthAccountsHistorical.

"CDC Sexually Transmitted Infection Costs (STIC) Figure and User's Manual." National Coalition of STD Directors. May 30, 2017. https://www.ncsddc.org/resource/cdc-sexually-transmitted-infection-costs-stic-figure-and-users-manual/.

"STI Treatment Guidelines Update." Sexually Transmitted Infections Treatment Guidelines, 2021, Centers for Disease Control and Prevention. https://www.cdc.gov/std/treatment-guidelines/default.htm.

Alexander, S. C. et al. "Sexuality Talk during Adolescent Health Maintenance Visits." *JAMA Pediatrics* 168, no. 2 (2014): 163–169. https://doi.org/10.1001/jamapediatrics.2013.4338.

Savoy, Margot, David O'Gurek, and Alexcis Brown-James. "Sexual Health History: Techniques and Tips." American Academy of Family Physicians, February 1, 2020. https://www.aafp.org/dam/AAFP/documents/journals/afp/Savoy.pdf.

Reno, Hilary, Ina Park, Kim Workowski, Aliza Machefsky, and Laura Bachmann. "A Guide to Taking a Sexual History." Centers for Disease Control and Prevention, 2015. https://www.cdc.gov/std/treatment/sexualhistory.pdf.

Levy, Andrea Gurmankin, Aaron M. Scherer, Brian J. Zikmund-Fisher, Knoll Larkin, Geoffrey D. Barnes, and Angela Fagerlin. "Prevalence of and

Factors Associated with Patient Nondisclosure of Medically Relevant Information to Clinicians." JAMA Netw Open. e185293. https://doi.org/10.1001/jamanetworkopen.2018.5293 November 30, 2018. https://jamanetwork.com/journals/jamanetworkopen/fullarticle/2716996.

*Farlex Partner Medical Dictionary*. S.v. "cypridophobia." Retrieved from https://medical-dictionary.thefreedictionary.com/cypridophobia.

### CHAPTER 9.
### Playing It Safe: An Ounce of Prevention

Khan, F., S. Mukhtar, I. K. Dickinson, and S. Sriprasad. "The Story of the Condom." *Indian Journal of Urology: IJU: Journal of the Urological Society of India* 29, no. 1. (2013): 12–15. https://doi.org/10.4103/0970-1591.109976.

Appler, Abigail Cline. "Put a Helmet on Your Privates Because They're Going to See Some Action: The History of Condoms in the Military." *Hektoen International, A Journal of Medical Humanities* 8, no. 4 (Spring 2017). https://hekint.org/2017/01/22/put-a-helmet-on-your-privates-because-theyre-going-to-see-some-action-the-history-of-condoms-in-the-military/#:~:text=As%20World%20War%20II%20began,use%20against%20sexually%20transmitted%20diseases.&text=European%20and%20Asian%20militaries%20on,civilian%20condom%20use%20in%201941.

"Fun Facts About Condoms!" Planned Parenthood, Condom Crawl. https://www.plannedparenthood.org/uploads/filer_public/54/38/5438b72e-82d6-4747-97bd-1a42c86d844c/fun_facts.pdf.

Choosing Wisely, an Initiative of the ABIM Foundation. https://www.choosingwisely.org/.

Burton, Taylor. "How Baby Boomers Will Impact the Future of Healthcare." Encompass Health. January 14, 2020. https://blog.encompasshealth.com/2020/01/14/how-baby-boomers-will-impact-the-future-of-healthcare/.

"STD Risk and Oral Sex—CDC Fact Sheet." Centers for Disease Control and Prevention. December 31, 2021. https://www.cdc.gov/std/healthcomm/stdfact-stdriskandoralsex.htm.

"What Are My Chances of Getting an STI?" STI Risk Chart. San Francisco City Clinic. https://www.sfcityclinic.org/patient-education-resources/std-risk-chart.

Joyal, Christian C., and Julie Carpentier. "The Prevalence of Paraphilic Interests and Behaviors in the General Population: A Provincial Survey." *Journal of Sex Research* 54, no. 2 (2017): 161–171. https://doi.org/10.1080/00224499.2016.1139034.

*The Diagnostic and Statistical Manual of Mental Disorders (DSM-V).* 5th ed. American Psychiatric Association Publishing, 2022.

Green, Emma. "Consent Isn't Enough: The Troubling Sex of Fifty Shades. The Blockbuster Fantasy Has Become a Big Movie—and a Bigger Problem." *The Atlantic.* February 10, 2015. https://www.theatlantic.com/culture/archive/2015/02/consent-isnt-enough-in-fifty-shades-of-grey/385267/.

Dean, Lucy. "Normal People: Bizarre Side Effect of Economic Downturn." Yahoo Finance. May 21, 2020. https://www.google.com/url?q=https://au.finance.yahoo.com/news/shoppers-purchase-erotica-sci-fi-during-economic-downturns-023810272.html&sa=D&source=docs&ust=1645111655545645&usg=AOvVaw3qkzSFm3HctblpNx6h5MBe.

Reagan, Courtney. "Bookstore Bonanza: The Economics of Erotica." Consumer Nation, CNBC. April 12, 2012. https://www.cnbc.com/2012/04/12/bookstore-bonanza-the-economics-of-erotica.html.

Aswell, Sarah. "1 in 5 of Your Friends Is Getting Kinky—Should You Be Too?" Healthline. Last Modified October 10, 2019. https://www.healthline.com/health/healthy-sex/kinky-sex-bdsm.

Castleman, Michael. "Orgies through the Ages: Today's Sex/Swing Clubs May Be on the Fringe, but They're Nothing New." *Psychology Today.* September 4, 2018. https://www.psychologytoday.com/us/blog/all-about-sex/201809/orgies-through-the-ages.

Rinard, Katherine, Thomas Nelius, LaMicha Hogan, Cathy Young, Alden E. Roberts, and Myrna L. Armstrong. "Cross-Sectional Study Examining Four Types of Male Penile and Urethral Play." *Ambulatory and Office Urology* 76, no. 6 (December 1, 2010): P1326–1333. https://doi.org/10.1016/j.urology.2010.03.080.

Leal, Samantha, and Emily Belfiore. "The 8 Best Kegel Balls for Everything from Better Sex to Incontinence." Health.com. November 11, 2021. https://www.health.com/sexual-health/kegel-balls.

"Size of the Sex Toy Market Worldwide from 2019 to 2026." Statista Research Department, Statista. February 2, 2022. https://www.statista.com /statistics/587109/size-of-the-global-sex-toy-market/.

"STI Treatment Guidelines Update." Sexually Transmitted Infections Treatment Guidelines, 2021, Centers for Disease Control and Prevention. Last modified July 22, 2021. https://www.cdc.gov/std/treatment-guidelines /default.htm.

"STD Diagnoses Among Key U.S. Populations, Five-Year Trends." Centers for Disease Control and Prevention. https://www.cdc.gov/nchhstp/newsroom /docs/factsheets/STD-Table-2018_Final.pdf.

## CHAPTER 10.
### Ready, Set, Sex

Nogoski, Emily. *Come As You Are: Revised and Updated: The Surprising New Science That Will Transform Your Sex Life*. New York: Simon & Schuster, 2021.

"Notes from the Field: Cluster of Lymphogranuloma Venereum Cases Among Men Who Have Sex with Men—Michigan, August 2015–April 2016." Centers for Disease Control and Prevention, *Morbidity and Mortality Weekly Report* 65, no. 34 (September 2, 2016): 920–921. https://www.cdc.gov /mmwr/volumes/65/wr/mm6534a6.htm.

"Zika and Pregnancy." Centers for Disease Control and Prevention, Women and Their Partners Trying to Become Pregnant, last modified March 24, 2021. https://www.cdc.gov/pregnancy/zika/women-and-their-partners .html.

"Transmission." Centers for Disease Control and Prevention, Ebola (Ebola Virus Disease), Last Modified January 14, 2021. https://www.cdc.gov/vhf /ebola/transmission/index.html.

"Dear Colleague Letter: DSTDP Lab and Drug Shortages" Centers for Disease Control and Prevention, Department of Health & Human Services, September 8, 2020. https://www.cdc.gov/std/general/DCL-Diagnostic -Test-Shortage.pdf.

Jameson, Marni. "Seniors' Sex Lives Are Up—and So Are STD Cases Around the Country." AARP, May 17, 2011. https://www.aarp.org/health

/conditions-treatments/news-05-2011/seniors_sex_lives_are_up_and_so
_are_std_cases.html.

Howley, Elaine K. "What to Know About Rising STD Rates Among Seniors."
*U.S. News*, Health. December 10, 2018. https://health.usnews.com/health
-care/patient-advice/articles/2018-12-10/what-to-know-about-rising-std
-rates-among-seniors.

# Index